P9-DEE-296

INCHES **OFF!**
Your Tummy

INCHES OFF!
Your Tummy

The Super-Simple **5-MINUTE PLAN**
to Firm Up Flab & Sculpt a Flat Belly

JORGE CRUISE

RODALE.

This book is intended as a reference volume only, not as a medical manual.
The information given here is designed to help you make informed decisions about your health.
It is not intended as a substitute for any treatment that may have been prescribed by your doctor.
If you suspect that you have a medical problem, we urge you to seek competent medical help.

The information in this book is meant to supplement, not replace, proper exercise training. All forms of exercise pose some inherent risks. The editors and publisher advise readers to take full responsibility for their safety and know their limits. Before practicing the exercises in this book, be sure that your equipment is well-maintained, and do not take risks beyond your level of experience, aptitude, training, and fitness. The exercise and dietary programs in this book are not intended as a substitute for any exercise routine or dietary regimen that may have been prescribed by your doctor. As with all exercise and dietary programs, you should get your doctor's approval before beginning.

Mention of specific companies, organizations, or authorities in this book does not imply endorsement by the author or publisher, nor does mention of specific companies, organizations, or authorities imply that they endorse this book, its author, or the publisher.

Internet addresses and telephone numbers given in this book were accurate at the time it went to press.

© 2013 by Jorge Cruise

All rights reserved. No part of this publication may be reproduced or transmitted in any form or by any means, electronic or mechanical, including photocopying, recording, or any other information storage and retrieval system, without the written permission of the publisher.

Rodale books may be purchased for business or promotional use or for special sales.
For information, please write to:
Special Markets Department, Rodale Inc., 733 Third Avenue, New York, NY 10017

Printed in the United States of America
Rodale Inc. makes every effort to use acid-free ♾, recycled paper ♻.

Photographs by Beth Bischoff
Book design by Elizabeth Neal

Library of Congress Cataloging-in-Publication Data is on file with the publisher.
ISBN 978-1-60961-497-3 paperback

Distributed to the trade by Macmillan
2 4 6 8 10 9 7 5 3 1 paperback

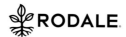

We inspire and enable people to improve their lives and the world around them.
rodalebooks.com

To the Rodale family:
Thank you for your belief
in me for the past 10 years.
Your support means
the world to me.

CONTENTS

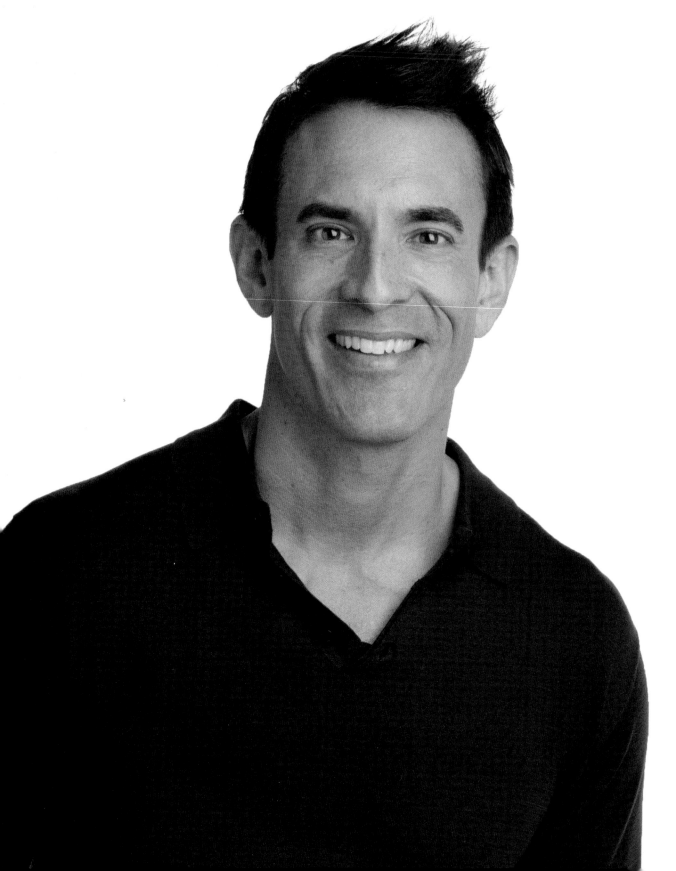

Welcome, Dear Friend.

What if everything we've been told about how to exercise our abs has been wrong? Crunches and situps, ab machines, and vibrating belts have become novelty items. So much so, that discussing how to get a nice midsection has become almost comedic, leading many to question the methods.

Science has shown that the secret to taking inches off your tummy in just 5 minutes a day is about doing the *right* strength-training exercises. This book will show you the precise combination of moves—primary exercise mixed with what I call active rest—making sure that your entire 5-minute routine is action packed and at an intensity that generates afterburn. By tapping into afterburn, along with your workout, you can burn up to 400 more calories in just 5 minutes a day.

Imagine melting off inches and burning up to 400 more calories in just 5 minutes each and every day—the reality is here!

LET'S GET MOVING.

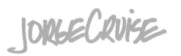

INTRODUCTION

I know what it's like to struggle with excess weight—I've lived it. I remember cringing after catching glimpses of myself in windows or mirrors and wanting to just hide away. I also remember always having to readjust my bunching tight clothes, how my belly would bulge over my pants, and how I always felt slow and out of breath. As a kid, gym class was humiliating: I was always picked last for any team and I couldn't even do a pushup—not a single one. Many people don't realize it, but I spent my formative years as the heavy kid in school. I tried every workout and diet out there to slim myself down, but I failed miserably every time.

By the ripe old age of 15, my health had already begun to deteriorate. I had headaches every day, I suffered from severe asthma, and I never had any energy. Surprisingly, no one ever suggested that these issues could have been linked to my diet and weight. But the more weight I gained, the less active I was, and my health issues became more frequent.

The worst part of being the fat kid in school was the rejection I felt. Kids are cruel, and they weren't shy about letting me know that I wasn't acceptable. Socially, doors close quickly and permanently when you're overweight. I was left with low self-esteem, insecurities, and depression.

I found my refuge at home. I grew up in Southern California with a loving family. My mom was from Mexico City and my dad was from Pennsylvania. My mother and grandmother came from the food-is-love school of parenting. We had incredible meals, both in serving size and deliciousness. I found pleasure in food and ate far too much. The reaction at home was approval. Food was love, after all, and I wanted so much to feel loved. And so a vicious cycle began—feel horrible and rejected in the outside world, feel loved and stuffed at home.

The beginning of the end of my struggle with weight happened when I was a teenager. I began to have nasty stomachaches in addition to the headaches and asthma I mentioned earlier. This went on for a few weeks, and when I was finally taken to the hospital, the doctors discovered a chunk of meat lodged in my appendix. I had to have emergency surgery to remove it.

That experience terrified me. I'd always thoughtlessly shoveled in whatever food was in front of me, and, besides hating the way I looked, I never considered what it was doing to my health. Later, after I learned the healthy way to lose weight and became more fit, my headaches and asthma went away, my energy surged, and so did my mood. Miracle cure? No. Just living a better lifestyle. And it's one you can have too.

But that's not the whole story.

When I turned 18, shortly after my hospital stay, my father was diagnosed with prostate cancer. I was scared. It just kept playing in my brain on an endless loop: "Dad has cancer." What I didn't know then, but would soon learn, was that some of the big risk factors for prostate cancer are a poor diet, excess weight, and lack of exercise.

I realized for the first time that I was on a very dangerous road, and so were the people I loved most. What did the future hold for me if I refused to change? I found motivation from my health crisis and my father's cancer. Together, my father and I remade our lifestyles. I was motivated so deeply to make a change, and to help those I loved, that I enrolled in college to study fitness and nutrition. It was the beginning of a lifelong quest to help myself and the people I love—all of you— find the path to freedom and happiness through optimal health and fitness.

So what does that mean for you?

You came to this book because you want to change your life. Well, I know exactly how it feels to want change badly, but not know how to get to that goal—I've been there. It took a pair of serious health scares to light a fire under me, and while it doesn't have to be that dramatic, you need to uncover your true inspiration.

The first key to losing inches is to find your deep emotional trigger—the one that will help you to truly pursue permanent, positive change in your life. I don't say this lightly; being deeply motivated is inherently necessary for long-lasting change, according to a wealth of scientific evidence and personal anecdotes from thousands of women and men I've helped over the years. If you want to change, you've got to find the emotional trigger that, when fired off, will light up your heart.

We all try with superficial triggers repeatedly: Bikini season approaches, a wedding is coming, or maybe it's time for your school's reunion—and you once again prepare to lose the weight. And maybe you drop 10 to 20 pounds, as

you've most likely done more than once in your lifetime, but then over the next several months the weight creeps back until you weigh more than you did to begin with. The deep, meaningful emotional trigger is the tipping point you need. For some, that trigger might be chest pains, a diabetes diagnosis, or a heart condition in yourself or someone you love. For others, it's watching lively children or grandchildren running and playing and knowing that if a change isn't made, you might not be around for the fun.

When you see people who have lost a lot of weight or reached some kind of major positive goal—an aunt, your best friend, the coworker down the hall—they've succeeded in part because they found that deep emotional trigger and pulled it. When you are profoundly motivated, failure stops being an option. To zero in on this, I want you to make a list (see the opposite page for specifics on how to do this). This will help you get beyond what I like to call magazine-cover motivators: I have a big event coming up; I want to fit into my "skinny" clothes; I want to look great naked. These are nice, but very few people find true lasting

SHARE YOUR **STORY!**

I want to hear why you've decided to take positive steps to change your life. I also want to hear about what great progress you're making. Share your story and interact with others just like you at:

facebook.com/jorgecruisefan

motivation in these things. Use your list to find your deep emotional triggers.

The second key to long-lasting change and a lifetime of fit and healthy living is having access to the right information and tools for successfully losing fat and inches. Obviously, it's great to be motivated, but without the right tools, you can't fix what's broken. The problem is that much of the conventional wisdom put forth by most fitness and weight-loss experts over the last

PULLING YOUR TRIGGER: PREPARING
UNBREAKABLE MOTIVATORS

Answer the big question: Why?

Why do you want to lose weight? Make a list. You may start off with things such as "look good for my class reunion," or "fit into my skinny jeans." Keep digging. What's the real reason you want to change? It's the deep emotional triggers that can keep you trudging the road to happy destiny when times get tough. You need to find that true, deep-down emotional trigger and use it to motivate you. This will create real conviction, as opposed to just "wanting to get in shape."

Ask yourself the following questions.

1. Who am I? Do my outsides match my insides? Am I who I want to be?

2. Why is being at a healthy weight and fit really important?

3. What is my mission? Who would benefit from my being healthier and happier?

4. What am I missing in my life? Energy? Happiness? Health?

5. What's my motivation for wanting to improve my food and exercise habits besides looking better?

6. What has caused me to fall off the wagon in the past? Are the obstacles still present? If so, how will I navigate them this time?

7. What am I doing in my life that's hurting me? Smoking? Drinking too much? Not exercising or eating right? Letting work interfere with relationships and health?

8. What do I truly need and want to feel whole? How is my current weight presenting an obstacle to what I really want in my life?

9. Am I happy? How would losing weight and becoming more fit make me happier inside?

Post your answers where you can see them to help you stay motivated over the following weeks and months. Grab some paper and write your answers.

Introduction

50 years has been, and still is, misguided—and just plain wrong. This is where I will set the record straight. In the following chapters I'll debunk erroneous guidelines for exercise and eating, and I'll provide you with the science that works with the way your body is made to function.

If you're holding this book in your hands, it means that you want to take inches off your tummy (and more!). I'm so happy you made the choice to change your life. That's what this book is all about: giving you the tools and knowledge you need to succeed and keeping you motivated and inspired to see your goals through.

The best part? You can reach your fitness goals *in just a few minutes a day!* As I mentioned in my welcome letter to you, my plan for fitness is guaranteed by science, and it works because it's designed for the way your body is biologically made to burn more calories and shed fat. The Inches Off! Your Tummy plan breaks down like this:

- In Chapters 1 and 2, I'll explain how health experts and government agencies have given misleading exercise recommendations that ultimately backfire, and I'll give specifics on the science that backs up my formula for success.

- In Chapters 3 and 4, we'll take action with the 4-week program. I'll describe how it works and what moves you'll do, plus give you options for other types of exercise you might enjoy.

- In Chapter 5, I'll break down the Inches Off! Your Tummy eating guidelines to help you reach your weight-loss goals even faster. This is effortless, delicious eating based on counting only the calories that cause weight gain. I'll also explain how you can prevent emotional eating and feel great about your relationship with food.

- In Chapter 6, I provide food lists that are calculated so you can easily track the calories that cause weight gain.

- In Chapter 7, I'll give you a peek into the future by discussing where you'll take the Inches Off! Your Tummy program after Week 4. Here you'll see how to ramp up your workouts, stay motivated for the long haul, and keep eating healthy in the weeks and months to come.

Okay, it's time to get moving! I can't wait for you to start this program. I promise, once you start losing inches and fat and gaining muscle and flexibility, everything will change. Your days will be brighter. You'll have more energy. And one day early on in the program, when you walk up a flight of stairs or carry in the groceries, you're going to realize, "Hey, this *is* easier," and that's just the beginning of the benefits. Yes, you're going to feel stronger and more energetic, but you're also going to sleep more restfully, feel happier and more serene, and you'll love the slim, sleek reflection that smiles back at you from the windows and mirrors that used to make you cringe.

Before we start, I want to leave you with one last thought: *Today counts more than yesterday or tomorrow.* Stay in the moment.

Keep that in mind no matter where you are in this program—or your life. Maybe you were overweight yesterday, but today change is afoot. Maybe you started this week strong, but yesterday you stumbled. Today you get up and keep moving forward. Maybe you're worried about a party that's coming up. Today you are creating the tools to deal with any challenge. It's a one-day-, one-moment-, one-breath-at-a-time philosophy.

Yesterday is history. Tomorrow doesn't exist. Today is the only day that matters.

MY TOP 10 BELIEFS
ABOUT HEALTH AND FITNESS

10. I believe the human body is designed for movement, not sofas.

9. I believe happiness is an attainable choice, not a right.

8. I believe exercise and intelligent eating are the cheapest, easiest, and healthiest paths to happiness and long life.

7. I believe that yesterday is history—no matter what happened—and today is an opportunity.

6. I believe emotional eating is one of the main reasons a person is fat.

5. I believe once you find your deep emotional trigger, change is easy.

4. I believe fear is one of the main reasons a person won't exercise.

3. I believe exercise, once you start, erases fear.

2. I believe anyone can sculpt the body he or she wants.

1. I believe in *you.*

Skip
Useless
Exercises
and Burn
400 More
Calories
per Day

"The first step towards getting somewhere is to decide that you are not going to stay where you are."

—J. P. MORGAN

One of my big beliefs is that the human body is designed to be active. But just to be crystal clear about the kind of activity I mean here, let me say that I'm not talking about running marathons, doing triathlons, deadlifting 300 pounds, or summiting Mount Everest—although those are all fantastic activities if they toot your horn. It's just that they aren't the sort of moving you need to do to lose inches off your body. All exercise is good, but the best workout is one you refuse to miss, and that's the type of movement I'm talking about. The problem is that the exercise recommendations given by most of the top health agencies won't keep you motivated because they don't deliver the results you're looking for.

THE FOLLY OF
CONVENTIONAL WISDOM

Most health experts recommend that you get an hour of moderate-level exercise or more a day—and this is just to maintain weight and improve health, not to lose fat or inches. While you'll often read that you can use exercise to lose weight, if you look closely at the majority of recommendations coming from the most valid sources, you'll see that they usually say some variation of "an hour of exercise most days of the week will prevent weight gain and improve health." Agencies that know their stuff, such as the American College of Sports Medicine and the American Council on Exercise, know that

the research doesn't back using exercise for weight loss, because it really doesn't work. At least, not the sort of daily exercise that is recommended. That's the biggest surprise in this whole picture: What these experts have told you, and are still telling you, about exercise, diet, and obesity won't give you the results you're looking for if you're trying to lose weight.

The sort of exercise that will shed fat and slim you down is the kind of exercise our ancestors did. To get in touch with this you need to understand how the human animal was made to live in its natural habitat.

MOVE WITH YOUR GENETIC BLUEPRINT—AND
SKIP USELESS EXERCISES

Our modern lifestyle is extremely foreign to the way our human bodies were designed to flourish—in fact, the way we live now accounts for only around 0.5 percent of our genetic history as humans. What accounts for the other 99.5 percent, around 2.5 million years, of our history was the time when we roamed the earth as hunter–gatherers. Back then, we were tribes of nomadic people who lived off the land—people who never heard of a remote control, let alone a couch. This is the type of living our bodies are wired to do.

Those of you who have read my previous books know that I often discuss the hunter–gatherers we used to be when it

REMEMBER YOUR
ANCESTORS

Whenever you feel like lying around and ignoring exercise, remember this: Inactivity is a new thing for humans. In fact, we've only been such sedentary creatures for a mere 0.5 percent of our genetic history. For more than 2 million years, or 99.5 percent of our history as humans, our ancestors spent their days foraging for food, hunting, and crossing great distances on foot. We humans were made to move our bodies—not sit on our behinds or go from point A to B in a motorized vehicle. Tap into this knowledge and personal power of locomotion. It's what we're made for. It's a gift. There are a lot of people out there who, because of injuries or other issues, *can't* move like you can—move for them. I try to keep this in mind whenever I'm having a low-energy day, and it motivates me to not take my ability to be active for granted. It helps me to remember that my body is a remarkable gift. So is yours. Don't waste your remarkable abilities; tap into your own personal power.

comes to eating habits (which I'll revisit to some extent in Chapter 5), and this same theory holds true for exercise.

Our ancestors did not struggle with excess weight, and they certainly didn't have an obesity epidemic on their hands. It's no coincidence that modern life and excess fat go hand in hand, but it's not just desk jobs, sofa-related leisure activities, automotive transportation (instead of walking), or 24/7 access to fast and unhealthy foods that are to blame. These factors do play a role, of course, but they aren't the central cause for why we can't get slim and healthy, despite what you hear from many agencies, including the World Health Organization, the Centers for Disease Control and Prevention, and the National Institutes of Health.

The way to stop doing *useless exercises (especially ab exercises)* that won't lead you toward your goals is to move the way our ancestors did. While studies show that our hunter–gatherer forebears didn't actually burn significantly more calories through exercise than the average modern human does, they did move a lot more throughout the day than we do today. This kind of movement wasn't regulated to walking for an hour on a treadmill or going to the gym three times a week to hoist weights for 20 to 45 minutes at a time. What our ancestors did was move in short bursts of intensity that would build muscle (hunters sprinted after animals or to keep from becoming prey, while gatherers dug for tubers, hoisted and carried the goods back to camp, and did so while carrying babies). Our forebears would also walk when necessary to get from one place to another, anywhere from 5 to 20 miles a day. When time allowed, they would sit. These people were lean and strong because they used their bodies in bursts of intense activity, intermixed with lots of low-level cardio and lots of resting too.

THE FORMULA FOR
SUCCESS

The Inches Off! Your Tummy program works with the way your body is biologically adapted to function—a 5-minute burst of energy and reasonable activity throughout the day—instead of making activity something you carve out hours for in the day. This is useful exercise because it gives your body just what it needs to build muscle and burn fat, which helps you shed inches quickly. This is my most effective and simple fitness and weight-loss program yet, and that's because working smarter is more important than working harder. I've compressed everything you need to optimize your returns—max calorie burn, max fat burn, minimal minutes. Most fitness plans keep you in a gym or in classes for hours each week, treadmilling your way through endless cardio quests or enduring heavy-handed training sessions with loud staffers pushing you to the breaking point. Reality TV glorifies this as well.

YOU ARE NOT
ALONE

Today, I'm well aware that my struggle is not an isolated one. Nearly two-thirds of the US population is either overweight or obese—that's more than 200 million people who have *billions* of pounds of excess fat dragging them down! And yes, we live in a society that encourages us to be this way: We are plagued by the 24/7 availability of foods that fatten us, sedentary desk jobs, and pastimes that involve moving only on laptop keyboards or remote controls. And the advice we've tried so hard to follow to cut calories, hit the gym, and move our bodies for 60 or even 90 minutes a day has all failed—but not for lack of trying. Most of us have tried to lose weight, and maybe even temporarily succeeded, only to have it return, and then some! The bottom line is that your inability to have the body you want isn't your fault. We tried to follow what the experts told us, and not that they were maliciously leading us in the wrong direction, but the fact is that we've all been led down a road to more fat.

You wonder how those fit people you see at the gym or running on the sidewalk got that way. Why aren't they fat? You probably blame yourself, like I did, but the reality is that you need the right tools to lose belly fat and keep it off. That's what this book is all about.

EXERCISE IS NOT **A FOUR-LETTER WORD**

How do you react when you hear the word *exercise*? Do you cringe, groan, or feel a flutter of anxiety?

That's okay. Exercise is a loaded word. We all know we're supposed to be more active. We hear it on TV, read it in magazines, and run it on a desperate loop in our own heads even if we don't lift a finger to do anything about it. We have friends and loved ones who take spinning classes, run road races, or rock climb. We see how they look—lean, healthy, full of energy. We know that they get those benefits from sweating regularly.

But despite all those benefits, the negative baggage we have surrounding exercise still hangs there in our minds. Exercise means time. Exercise means work. Exercise means discomfort.

Sometimes the hardest thing in the world is getting past that word, exercise, and lacing up your sneakers to get the job done. I understand that. I've coached millions of people. And I've also coached the worst client in exercise history: myself.

Of course I have days—more than a few, honestly—when I feel glued to my sheets, when the thought of rising into the sunshine and working up a sweat makes me moan and bury my head under the pillow.

Then I think about what I know deep in my bones.

- **I KNOW** I'll feel better once I get moving.

- **I KNOW** I'll feel better still when I enter the zone, that time during my workout when I feel stronger than I did the day before.

- **I KNOW** I'll feel best of all when I'm finished, smiling, looking forward to a great day because I'm energized and proud of myself.

But there's something else. Something I know that's even more motivating and enticing than all those good feelings I just listed.

- **I KNOW,** because of my experience and what research shows, that I don't have to exercise for hours and hours each week to keep myself fit and reach my goals.

Welcome to a new way to work out.
Welcome to my 5-Minute Fitness Formula.

That's why I designed Inches Off! the way I did—to work with the way your body was made to operate biologically, while also being quick and efficient for the modern human in all of us—so you won't want to skip my workouts. I don't have a put-in-the-hours philosophy. My approach is incredibly effective and based on three components:

1. **THE PHYSICAL.** You will move the way your body was made to move.

2. **THE NUTRITIONAL.** You will eat the way your body was made to eat.

3. **THE EMOTIONAL.** You will identify the emotional triggers that will make positive change easier.

The result: You'll burn up to 400 more calories per day, and you'll lose inches off your belly by using my program—and the best part is that it will only take you 5 minutes of carved-out exercise time per day. This is not useless exercise; this is a fitness plan that zeros in on exactly what your body needs.

A typical 5-minute routine can burn anywhere from 30 to 40 calories. Let me share with you how you can burn up to 400 calories in the same amount of time by using the science of the Inches Off! workouts.

First, it's important to understand

CARDIO COMPLEMENTS **YOU**

After reading this chapter, you might think I'm against traditional cardio workouts. Not a chance! I support and encourage any and every form of exercise. The fact is our society doesn't move enough—period. Whatever keeps people active and working up a sweat is just fine with me. And moving your body outside of my 5-minute formula is something I recommend—with a caveat or two. Cardio won't build muscle or help you lose weight directly. However, that said, including a 20- to 30-minute easy walk, fun family bike ride, dancing around your living room session, or swim can help you stick to your other goals better. Here's how:

Longer, more moderate and steady exercise, especially when done outside and/or with friends or family, boosts chemical messengers in your body (neurotransmitters and hormones) that improve your mood, increase energy, and lower stress. The key is to make sure that any additional exercise is fun, relaxing, and moderate.

that after any exercise session your body raises its calorie-burning engine to replace the work you've just done; you take in more oxygen, you repair and build muscles, and your body does cellular work to remove toxins built up during exercise—this is afterburn. The more intense the exercise, the more you alternate the intensity (intervals), and the more you build muscle, the more calories your body burns. In a new groundbreaking study, researchers from the University of Colorado found that exercisers burned up to 200 more calories per day by doing just 2.5 minutes of exercise. The study had its subjects perform high-intensity sprints on stationary bicycles and then tracked their calorie burn for the next 24 hours. The reason for the elevated calorie burning? Afterburn.

Second, muscle burns more calories than fat. While this fact is widely accepted, the amount of calories burned by muscle is still up for debate, but the range has been placed at 30 to 100 calories per day per pound of muscle (in comparison, 1 pound of fat burns about 3 calories a day). Since I stick with the latest findings, I can comfortably say that a pound of muscle burns about 35 calories a day. For example, in two studies, one published by the *American Journal of Clinical Nutrition* and the other by the *Journal of Applied Physiology*, researchers found that you can burn an extra 35 calories a day for each

pound of muscle you gain. That might not sound like much, but you can potentially gain 4 pounds of slim, sleek muscle and drop the same amount or more of fat during the next 4 weeks with my program—that adds up to an extra 140 calories burned off each day, while you are doing nothing!

Finally, the type of workout you do accounts for a higher calorie burn during the workout as well as after your exercise session. Based on available research, it is clear that the best way to get both is through combining intervals (different intensities of moving) with muscle-fatiguing strength moves that work several muscles at once. This also is how your body was genetically designed to move. I based my 5-Minute Fitness Formula on this research and similar scientific studies that looked at comparable high-intensity interval training regimens that also show increased calorie burning in the 24 to 48 hours after short-duration, high-intensity workouts. With my exercises you'll maximize your calorie-burning potential so you shave off inches and belly fat quickly—in just a few minutes a day.

"HOW CAN ANYONE GET AMAZING RESULTS BY EXERCISING ONLY 5 MINUTES A DAY?"

That's the real question, isn't it? The next chapter will answer this question by showing you the science behind what makes my kind of exercise philosophy the most effective. You'll learn how my 5-Minute Fitness Formula will be applied for the next 4 weeks, and I'll describe what kind of exercise you'll be doing and why it is the key to losing inches from your tummy.

TWO GOOD REASONS PEOPLE EXERCISE FOR
AN HOUR OR MORE A DAY

I'm not against long workouts and high-volume exercise programs. But they have to be appropriate for you. For most people, it's just not useful. Here are two situations where long workouts would work for you.

1. YOU HAVE A SPECIFIC ATHLETIC GOAL.
People who exercise more than an hour a day are usually pushing toward a specific objective: completing a marathon, half-marathon, or triathlon; competing in a sport (football, basketball, etc.); or hitting bodybuilding/power-lifting goals.

A performance goal is a great thing, and it keeps thousands of people out there working hard and feeling great. If that's you—awesome. But if not, less exercise, not more, is probably the best approach.

2. YOU LOVE IT LIKE CRAZY.
Some people fall in love with certain forms of exercise: running, cycling, tennis, yoga, Pilates, weight training. Maybe they do it with friends as a social activity. But on some basic level, they simply love doing it.

Again, if that's you—awesome. I just ask you to check in on how you feel after your activity. If you have plenty of energy, great, but if you find that you drag throughout the rest of the day, then you may want to look at modifying your hobby by doing it fewer days a week or shortening the time frame.

Chapter

2

The
5-Minute
Fitness
Formula
Guaran-
teed by
Science

"They always say time changes things, but you actually have to change them yourself."

—ANDY WARHOL

How can I promise you results in just 5 minutes a day? Thanks to new research into the best exercise for shaving inches off your body and revving up your calorie burn, we now know that it only takes minutes a day of the right sort of exercise to get results. First, let's take a look at how your body burns fat. Normally when a woman loses weight, she loses 75 percent as fat, but up to 25 percent as muscle as well! Not with my Inches Off! Your Tummy design. That's because it focuses on strength training (also known as resistance training), which builds muscle, and muscle tissue uses fat for its fuel. That means for every new pound of muscle you add, you will shed more body fat—and this increased burn even remains revved at nighttime when you are sleeping. So instead of burning, say, 60 calories of fat per hour, you can burn twice that—up to 120 calories per hour or more—by adding muscle to your body. And don't worry about bulk. Many women still fear that adding muscle adds bulk to their bodies—but actually the opposite is true. Muscle sits more compactly on your body, so you look leaner and you lose inches—even if the scale doesn't budge. If you compare the mass of 5 pounds of fat to 5 pounds of muscle, you will see how much less in appearance there really is—about one-third the size.

5-MINUTE FITNESS FORMULA WORKS

In a word: intensity. My 5-Minute Fitness Formula is designed to be more intense and more efficient than most ordinary 20- to 30-minute gym workouts. It's that simple. I've taken the best findings in exercise science for shedding fat and losing inches and combined them to provide you with superior results.

The first component is called **high-intensity interval training**, or HIIT (this is a short-duration, high-intensity interval workout). An interval is a period of time when you exercise at a higher intensity; between intervals is the time you rest or move at a much less intense rate. For many workouts, this pace allows you to do more repetitions of an exercise in a shorter period of time. A typical HIIT workout is far shorter than, say, your garden-variety, 30-minute, one-speed-fits-all treadmill session.

What makes Inches Off! superior to other high-intensity interval workouts is that it challenges virtually every muscle in your body nonstop for the entire 5 minutes, so not only are you working at a heart-pumping intensity, you are building muscle from head to toe. All of this equals maximum calorie burn during your workout, and elevated calorie burn for the 24 hours after your workout—up to 400 more calories! And 5 minutes is a good time period because it's long enough and intense enough to give you real results, and short enough that you won't feel beat up for the rest of the day.

So how can my workout hit virtually every muscle in your body for 5 minutes straight? That brings us to the second component: **compound exercises**. That's a fancy way of saying you'll do exercises that combine multiple movements to work multiple muscle groups at the same time.

Sound complicated? It's not. Think of it this way: If you pick up light dumbbells and do a basic bicep curl, you're working your biceps, a few other arm muscles, and that's about it.

But if you do a forward lunge holding those same dumbbells, add a torso twist while curling them, and then press your arms over your head as you lunge, well, in the same amount of time as that bicep curl, you work your arms, shoulders, back, abdominals, hips, glutes, and every other muscle in both legs.

Add it all up: If you do a series of compound exercises nonstop for 5 minutes at different intensities, you compress an entire workout's worth of head-to-toe fat burning into one short but comprehensive total-body workout.

That's intense. That's efficient. That's why the 5-Minute Fitness Formula works.

So why are shorter workouts that include intervals (high-intensity bursts of activity) so much more effective? I discussed this to some extent in the beginning of the book, but researchers who study interval training also speculate that:

- More intense workouts tell your body that you need to burn stored fat at a higher rate than steady-state cardio. In short, more intensity burns more fat.

- Intense training can release more growth hormones after a workout; growth hormones are chemical messengers that, when released into the bloodstream, tell your body it needs to repair and build more fat-burning muscle. Muscle tissue burns more calories, pound for pound, than fat tissue, even when you are not working out.

- Interval training increases your body's afterburn. This is the fancy word experts and fitness buffs like to use for the increased calorie burning you'll see after you do an interval workout. Afterburn refers to the fact that after an interval workout, your body burns calories at an elevated rate for up to 24 hours. This is most technically referred to as excess postexercise oxygen consumption, and it happens with steady-state exercise too, but at a lower rate. Afterburn happens because the more oxygen your body consumes, the more calories you burn, even after you're done exercising. As mentioned earlier, groundbreaking research from the University of Colorado found that exercisers burned up to 200 more calories a day after doing just 2.5 minutes of high-intensity interval training. Remember, we are doing 5 minutes of exercise that will match this—so by the end of 4 weeks you could be burning up to 400 more calories a day.

WHY THE 5-MINUTE FITNESS FORMULA
MELTS BELLY FAT FIRST

Here's the most exciting part and why this book is titled *Inches Off! Your Tummy*: These types of workouts tend to burn belly fat first.

When we hear about losing fat, most of us don't realize that the body has more than one type of fat. We actually have two, and when it comes to weight loss, shedding inches, and improving your health, it matters.

Visceral fat. This is fat that collects in and around your vital organs (your viscera = visceral). This is toxic fat. It interferes with the function of your most important organs like your liver and pancreas. It can also lead to metabolic syndrome, insulin resistance, and type 2 diabetes—which in turn can lead to heart attack and stroke. This is classic belly fat, and it's nasty stuff.

Subcutaneous fat. This is fat stored below your skin, closer to the surface. Saddlebags and big booties are caused by subcutaneous fat. This fat isn't as life threatening as visceral fat, but it's not something most of us like.

It's long been said that women can have different body shapes depending on how they store excess fat. Visceral fat gives you an apple shape. Subcutaneous fat gives you the pear. But I'll be honest: Chances are, even if you're a pear, you probably have some visceral fat to go with it. Folks can even be considered skinny-fat, where they don't look overweight, per se, but they have a little potbelly that's all visceral fat.

Visceral fat is the most dangerous when it comes to your health. Luckily, our bodies operate with some intelligence, and visceral fat is usually the first fat to be burned when you begin an exercise program.

Why? Well, think of your body like a building that is heated by a furnace. Your belly is your furnace, and that's where the majority of the metabolic work is done. That's the area of the body where food is digested, blood sugar is regulated, energy is burned, and excess energy is stored as fat for later. In a building, this would be the furnace. When you stoke up that furnace—firing up your metabolism with

(continued on page 14)

THE BENEFITS OF
INCREASING MUSCLE MASS

A lot of women avoid resistance training because they don't want to bulk up, but that's a huge myth. You'd have to lift incredibly heavy weights and eat large amounts of food to bulk up like a power lifter or bodybuilder would. Using resistance—through body weight, weights, or resistance bands—is one of the keys to building the lean, toned body you want. Here are just a few direct benefits of resistance training.

- **MORE STRENGTH.** Tasks that you used to dread—such as bringing in the groceries, taking out the trash, cleaning the house—might still not feel fun, but they will feel easier, and you'll have more energy to do them.

- **BETTER DAY-TO-DAY FUNCTIONING.** Everyday activities like climbing stairs, getting out of your car, or lifting a new box of laundry soap or cat litter will be easier. As a result, life becomes easier.

- **ALL-DAY CALORIE BURN.** The muscle you're going to build will help you burn more fat, and the daily exercises will increase your body's calorie-burning engine even when you are not exercising. Combined with the eating tips in Chapter 5, this can help you burn up to 400 calories more every day.

- **MORE EFFECTIVE BLOOD SUGAR MANAGEMENT.** Muscle helps process blood sugar, so adding muscle can help your body manage glucose and insulin. I'll discuss this more in Chapter 5, but know this: The higher your blood sugar, the higher your insulin—and the higher your insulin, the more your body stores and hangs on to stubborn belly fat.

- **JOINT STABILITY.** Muscles support joints, from your knees to your back. The more support a joint has, the less chance it has of giving you pain. This is important for improving or preventing osteoarthritis pain or common lower-back pain.

- **BETTER WORKOUTS.** Muscle begets muscle. The stronger you get, the better your workouts, which makes you even stronger. It's a positive cycle.

- **MORE FUN.** Personal relationships will improve, whether you're talking about being outside and active with loved ones, higher levels of happiness and laughter, or even more desire for intimacy in the bedroom (yes, I just told you that sex will be better).

- **A PSYCHOLOGICAL BOOST.** Exercise is a proven natural antidepressant that has been shown to work as effectively as medication and therapy. My workout will also boost your self-esteem, confidence, and positive outlook on life.

If that's not enough—check out the list below for other benefits you'll gain from my Inches Off! Your Tummy workouts.

- Increases bone density
- Improves balance and agility
- Lowers blood pressure
- Decreases bad cholesterol; increases good cholesterol
- Lowers the risk of stroke, diabetes, cancer, and arthritis
- Reduces insomnia; improves sleep
- Protects against illness

high-intensity exercise—you make it burn hotter. That's your body using energy.

Now, every furnace needs fuel. So where would you store that fuel? Six stories away in another part of the building? No. An old-school furnace would have the big coal bin right there next to it. Similarly, your body tends to burn the fuel that's closest—either food you've recently eaten or the excess energy that's been stored as fat. And visceral fat is **right there** in and around your metabolic center, liver, pancreas, etc. Your body burns that first.

That's a big reason why subcutaneous fat areas—better known as your trouble zones (your thighs, butt, and "granny arms")—can be so hard to slim down. The fat stored here is like excess energy stored for a rainy day by your body, but it's been stored the equivalent of those six stories away in another part of the building. Your body will get to it eventually—and will even burn some at the same time it burns the visceral fat. But when the visceral fat goes, that's when you lose inches off your tummy.

THE SCIENCE BEHIND THE
5-MINUTE FITNESS FORMULA

Many researchers have done studies on low-volume interval training (think short, intense workouts) compared to high-volume, steady-state cardio training (think long runs or treadmill sessions at one steady pace). The research universally shows that short, intense workouts are equally or more effective for burning fat, revving energy, and losing inches.

For example, in a 2006 study published in the *Journal of Physiology,* researchers found that a short-duration interval routine had the same physical effect as a long-lasting endurance workout. The interval group exercised for about 10 minutes per session, with more than half of that being rest time, while the steady-exercise people moved for 45 or more minutes for each workout. At the end of 2 weeks, both groups showed similar gains in fitness. Which would you choose?

Other research has shown that sedentary people who have low aerobic capacity (meaning that they can't exercise for long periods) have a higher risk for diseases including heart disease, stroke, and diabetes, as well as other health issues. This isn't surprising news, of course, but maybe this is: High-intensity interval training, like the kind described in the paragraph above, has been shown to have a greater effect on decreasing markers of disease and improving fitness than longer, more moderate exercise. Similar findings have been shown in people with no elevated risk for disease or health problems, as well as folks with serious health issues like heart failure, high cholesterol, excess weight, obesity, diabetes, and stroke.

How about fat loss? Intervals are superior here too. You've probably heard that people who do long, steady workouts (running or biking, for example) get into the fat-burning zone and blast more fat during their workouts. Actually, intervals seem to be superior, according to studies that have repeatedly shown that short-duration, high-intensity interval workouts produce a substantially greater calorie and fat burn. One study in the journal *Metabolism* compared two groups—one doing steady-state moderate exercise and the other doing shorter, more intense intervals. The interval group lost nine times more fat!

ONE LAST ARGUMENT ON
WHY LESS IS MORE

You'll never hear me bash any sort of exercise. Ever. But you need to know why there is such a thing as too much exercise, and that too much, or the wrong sort of activity, may not give you the benefits you think it will—for a number of reasons.

Recently, a Danish study followed three groups of sedentary men. (The researchers believe that their findings are applicable to women as well.) The first group maintained their activity level (that would be, none); the second group exercised for 30 minutes a day; and the third group exercised for 60 minutes a day (all workouts were steady state; no intervals). At the end of 3 months, the no-exercise group had lost no weight. The hour-long workout group lost 5 pounds each, on average. But the 30-minute group? These folks averaged a weight loss of **7 pounds each.**

How can that be? How can a group that exercised twice as much as another lose less weight? Well, it's counterintuitive, but here are the main reasons that longer workouts can backfire on you.

The more you exercise, the more you eat. Long workouts burn a lot of calories, so your body craves more food—not just to fuel the workout, but also to help it recover afterward. Yes, your body will have a legitimate nutritional need for more food, but **that's the trap.** Our bodies are designed to maintain balance: If you burn off a large number of calories, your body works hard to replace this energy by making you hungrier. Unfortunately, it is far too easy to replace the 300 or so calories you just burned off in an hour—one moderately portioned turkey sandwich (hold the mayo) and you're done. Often people mistakenly think that they can go hog wild after a workout that feels like a real bear. Using the "I need more fuel" or the "I deserve it" mentality, you might treat yourself to a Starbucks Caramel Frappuccino, and there goes 410 calories—it really doesn't take much.

Unless you swim like Michael Phelps, who burns somewhere around 12,000 calories a day (and even he has a personal nutrition coach who measures exactly what his body needs), it's likely that longer workouts can lead you to overeat.

The rest of your day is shot. The participants in the previous study also wore electronic sensors that measured their activity 24 hours a day, not just when they were exercising. The longest-duration exercisers tended to be far less active during the rest of their day. Maybe they felt too tired or possibly they felt a sense of entitlement about the rest of the day, thinking that they deserved to take it easy because of the workout. Other research demonstrating that people compensate by expending less energy to offset calories burned during exercise backs this theory up. The moderate exercisers, on the other hand, were more active and had more energy for the rest of the day's activities. This is the zone I want you to be in.

I want you living an active life beyond the Inches Off! workouts. I want you energetic, feeling good, and optimistic. I want the 5-Minute Fitness Formula to be a gateway to your amazing day, not the center of it.

THE BENEFITS

You'll get the following benefits on the Inches Off! Your Tummy program.

1. You'll build muscle.

HOW? Resistance training—working muscles against an outside force such as a band or weight—damages existing muscle, which is a good thing. When your body repairs the muscle, it will be sleeker and stronger. Remember, muscle will not bulk you up; it will slim you down.

2. You'll improve cardiovascular fitness.

HOW? Doing compound exercises for 5 minutes without rest will make you breathe hard, which improves your heart and lung health, revs your calorie-burning engine, and makes you stronger.

3. You'll raise your all-day metabolism.

HOW? Muscle is an amazing substance. It not only gives you strength, it's metabolically active tissue that burns calories just by existing. So the more muscle you build, the more calories your body will burn—up to 400 a day.

ARE YOU READY TO
BURN SOME FAT?

By now, I hope you can see why my 5-Minute Fitness Formula can help you transform your body—and life. I'm a big-time realist. In today's world, people don't have a lot of time for long workouts. The time you have to exercise should be used to its utmost potential. Workouts need to be fast, effective, and efficient.

Luckily, continuing research has helped show us the way. Short, intense workouts can be more effective than long, slow slogs. Now it's time to get started with the 5-Minute Fitness Formula. In the next chapter, you'll see how the next 4 weeks will lay out for you. I've set the plan up for incredible convenience and simplicity. You'll get detailed photos and instructions for each exercise, how long you need to do them, and how often. I can say with total honesty that it's one of the best workout programs I've ever created. I expect you to see and feel results in as little as a week.

Sound good?

Let's get going!

SPECIAL CASES

While almost everyone can benefit from an exercise program like *Inches Off! Your Tummy*'s, there are instances where caution is called for.

IF YOU HAVEN'T EXERCISED IN A LONG TIME—or have never exercised—check with your doctor before starting. Exercise is one of the healthiest things you can do for yourself, but it's always a good idea to find out if you have any underlying medical reasons not to start this program. Trust me, your doctor will be glad to see you when you say you want to start exercising. It's best to be safe.

IF YOU'RE PREGNANT, please consult your doctor before starting any exercise program. Pregnancy brings on a host of changes in your body, increasing your need for a number of nutrients and making some types of exercise—especially those that involve lying on your back—dangerous for you and your baby.

Chapter

3

The
4-Week
Inches
Off! Your
Tummy
Program

"You are never too old to set another goal or to dream a new dream."

—C. S. LEWIS

YOUR SUPER-SIMPLE
4-WEEK PLAN

This is your plan based on the 5-Minute Fitness Formula. This plan is simple, it's fun, and if you follow it faithfully, you'll burn up to 400 more calories per day, lose inches, feel more energized, and be happier!

I've made the Inches Off! Your Tummy program as easy as possible to follow and understand. The exercises may be new to you, but no worries, I've included descriptive photos, detailed instructions, and modifications in the next chapter so you can make any move work for your fitness level. Plus, you won't need to go to a gym (unless you want to), and you don't have to do any additional exercise outside of the 5 minutes you'll need to set aside for the workouts. That said, I will discuss the addition of fun and carefree cardio, if desired, to help you feel even better and get to your goals even faster. The process is easy.

WORKOUT
OVERVIEW

Each day (except Sundays) you'll do the following:

1. Run through the 5-minute workout.

2. Follow the Inches Off! eating plan all day, starting on page 152.

3. Foam-roll your muscles for a few minutes in your spare time (see the next chapter).

It's that easy.

Yes, I know that me saying it's easy is, well . . . easy. But truly, all you have to invest is minutes a day. These workouts are short, so you will never feel like it's impossible to fit them in, no matter how crazy your schedule. You may feel some soreness, but it will be a good sore that tells you your muscles are getting stronger and burning more calories. You'll also feel energized afterward and more awake for the rest of the day, so those 5 minutes you give up will actually give you more hours back in your day.

I often recommend that my clients do their exercises first thing in the morning. Research has shown that exercising muscles in the morning can help raise your metabolism for the rest of the day. A morning workout also launches you into your day with a positive mind-set. But in reality, you can do these workouts anytime. At lunch, it will break up your day and boost your afternoon energy levels. In the evening, you can do them while watching TV. You pick the most convenient time for yourself . . . *but you must do them*. No workout, no results.

WHAT EQUIPMENT WILL YOU **NEED?**

A gym will have all of this equipment. But if you want to outfit your own home gym, you can do it for a couple hundred dollars. Most items fit under a bed or in a closet, and some are ideal for travel, so you'll never have to miss a workout on the road.

Medicine ball ($20–50)
These come in various shapes, weights, and styles. Some have handles molded into the sides, which makes the ball much easier to hold or use as a base for floor exercises.

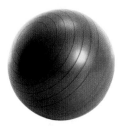

Swiss ball ($40–50)
This large, inflatable rubber ball is used for support in certain exercises. It's designed to force smaller stabilizing muscles to fire, giving you a more effective workout.

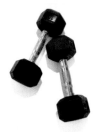

Dumbbells ($5–20, depending on weight)
These also come in various weights and styles (some are plain-old iron and others are coated with colorful rubber). I recommend using hexagonal (6-sided) dumbbells, which have flat sides. These are safer to use as a base for floor exercises. Round dumbbells can roll. Also: Always buy in pairs!

Sliders/gliders ($20–30)
These are flat plastic discs you can use to slide on different floor surfaces. On carpeting, a paper plate can work as well.

Resistance bands ($10–35; some come as a multiband kit)
These are like big rubber bands. Some have handles on either end, and some are circular bands. They can add resistance to a variety of exercises and fit in any overnight bag (a gym in your suitcase!).

THE COMPONENTS OF THE **5-MINUTE FITNESS ROUTINE**

For each workout, you'll have two exercises. You can't get much simpler than that, right? Here's how they break down.

- **PRIMARY EXERCISE.** The technical name for this is "complex," but these exercises aren't complex at all. This just means they involve more than one movement and more than one muscle group. These are the exercises that will work virtually your entire body at once.

- **ACTIVE REST.** This is a simpler, *secondary* exercise you perform while taking a break from the primary exercise.

The 5-minute workout alternates between primary exercise and active rest each minute for 5 minutes. Like so:

- **60 SECONDS: PRIMARY EXERCISE**

- **60 SECONDS: ACTIVE REST**

- **60 SECONDS: PRIMARY EXERCISE**

- **60 SECONDS: ACTIVE REST**

- **60 SECONDS: PRIMARY EXERCISE**

5 minutes and you're done!

DON'T BREAK **FORM**

As you do the exercises in this plan, it's important that you maintain proper form. If you get tired and start to break form, you could injure yourself. So here's what I recommend.

- Follow the exercise descriptions.

- Use a mirror if you have access to one (gyms will have them, but at home, any floor mirror will do). Also, a friend or exercise partner can watch you.

- Work with only as much weight as you can without breaking form.

- If you're working with body weight only, go as fast as you can without breaking form. It's more important to do fewer proper reps than more sloppy ones.

- Work at your own pace. If you must rest, only take as much time as you need. Don't worry—you'll get stronger!

SOME HELPFUL
HINTS

As you start this new program, I have some tips that will help you as you go. I use these strategies myself, and they keep me fired up and positive even when I know I'm going to have a crazy-busy day.

- **GO AT YOUR OWN PACE.**
These are timed workouts. As I like to say, "5 minutes and you're done!" This allows you to control your workout intensity. If you need to slow down, you can. If you feel strong and want to go harder, do it. No matter your pace, "5 minutes and you're done!"

- **THINK OF THIS AS PLAYTIME.**
Yes, they're called "work" outs. But you're doing them to look and feel better. Human bodies are designed to move. It's all positive. So think of this short window of time as playtime. It's your time to play, just for you and no one else.

- **ASK THE RIGHT QUESTIONS.**
I call them results-driven questions. Think of it this way: If you ask yourself questions in a negative way, you'll always be distracted by the negative. So always lean toward the positive. Instead of asking yourself, "Why is it so difficult for me to lose

THE MOTIVATOR USE YOUR WORDS!

If you're not in the same shape as your athletic friends, a favorite celebrity, or a professional athlete, you can get caught up in a word trap. Maybe you think those other people have more "talent," better "genetics," or easier access to "trainers" than you do. But those aren't the key words that matter. You're tougher than you think. How do I know? I was once overweight and out of shape, and I've worked with thousands of women and men who have shared this same struggle. I know for a fact that "talent" is overrated. The biggest challenges in life are more mental than physical. Instead, try on one of the following words:

Determination   **Tenacity**   **Drive**   **Inspiration**
Courage   **Resolve**   **Motivation**

These are *your* words. Focus your mind on the positive in yourself and you can reach your goals.

weight?" ask: "What can I do today to help me achieve my goal?" President Abraham Lincoln put it best: "People are just as happy as they make up their minds to be."

WHAT ABOUT **REST?**

You'll notice that the workouts don't mention rest. That's deliberate. I'd like you to try doing each workout without any rest in between exercises (besides the time it takes you to set up for the next exercise). These 5-minute workouts are designed to be short and intense. As you read earlier, interval workouts are incredibly effective. I want you breathing hard (cardio); I want your muscles to feel a burn (muscle building). I want you to have a terrific total-body workout in a very short time.

So here's what I recommend: Try to go without rest. If you need rest during or in between exercises, take it, but only the minimum you need. Push yourself! Remember the goal: Five minutes and you're done!

You can do this. You're stronger than you think, and you'll amaze yourself.

TAKE SUNDAY **OFF**

If you want rest, you can have a whole day! Sunday should be your time to recharge and think about how well you did the previous week and how fired up

SIMPLIFY? OR **SUPERCHARGE?**

For the primary exercises in the 5-minute workouts, you'll see additional instructions that tell you how to simplify or supercharge them. You don't have to do either. You can do the exercises as written and get great results. But I include these additional options to allow for greater flexibility, depending on your fitness level and athletic ability. Here's what I mean.

SIMPLIFY IT: Some of the following exercises have multiple movements that involve multiple body parts. That's the nature of compound exercises. If an exercise is too complex or too difficult for you in the early days of the program, feel free to simplify the exercise per the instructions. You'll still get great results, and you can perform the regular version as you make gains.

SUPERCHARGE IT: If you're feeling strong as you do an exercise, use these instructions to add a little something extra to the move—a supercharged version. If you're able to graduate to the supercharged version as you move through the program, you know you're seeing solid strength and flexibility gains. Keep going!

you'll be next week. You don't have to have a formal workout on Sunday, but I think getting out and being active is a great thing. Go for a walk with friends or family (or a dog). If it's warm, hit the neighborhood pool. Go for a bike ride.

The point of Sunday is to reset, recharge, reboot—but not just your body, your mind too. Enjoying yourself and your active life is one of the best ways to do that. Have some fun!

"SHOULD I DO **MORE?**"

After 5 minutes, you may wonder if you should do more. You may feel like you *want* to do more. I encourage you! The fact is you can get the results you want with the 5-Minute Fitness Formula and proper eating. But if you want to be even more active, go for it. Maybe you'll want to walk, run, or bike with friends later in the day. Do it! Maybe your sister-in-law will invite you to a fitness class before the kids get home from school. Have fun!

My only caveat is this: Listen to your body. How do you feel? Are your muscles fatigued? If you haven't been regularly active before trying the 5-Minute Fitness Formula, that workout alone will probably be plenty. Try to do more if you like, but I would much rather have you be able to do this program each day without skipping a day because you overdid it with extra activity the day before.

This also goes for the 5-minute workouts themselves. If you feel like you've overworked a muscle or if something hurts or feels off, back off and take a rest. (Also, see the box on foam rollers starting on page 144—they are a great way to get a self-massage for sore, tight muscles.) Most muscle aches and pains improve in a few days, but if you have joint pain, you should have it checked out by a doctor, preferably a sports doctor. Ordinary muscle soreness is to be expected—don't sweat that. But concentrated pain is a different thing. Again, listen to your body.

THE MOTIVATOR COUNT IT ALL UP AND SAY, "WOW!"

The 5-Minute Fitness Formula is only one small part of your day. Tonight before bed, tally up in your mind all the activity you did during the day: your regular exercises, plus climbing several flights of stairs, walking the dog, lifting those laundry baskets and grocery bags. Think of all the steps you took and all the muscles you worked. Not bad, right? Feel pretty jazzed about tomorrow morning, right?

ONE FINAL **NOTE**

I'll give you one last thing to think about before you start. You'll see that this is a 4-week plan with a different set of exercises each day (except Sunday, your rest day). At the end of 4 weeks, you'll feel great. You'll feel different. But I hope you won't feel done. I hope you go right back to the "Day 1" section in this chapter and start another 4 weeks. You'll feel like a pro and do the exercises that much better, with that much more strength and flexibility. You'll be able to do more reps in the allotted time. You'll continue to gain (and lose!).

Okay, it's time to start exercising. Have fun, feel great, and get ready to drop inches off your tummy!

WORKOUT WEEKS

1-2

AT A GLANCE

Here you'll find the exercises listed for each week. Detailed descriptions and photos for all moves are in the next chapter.

Week 1

Day 1	Day 2	Day 3
60 SECONDS: Squat and Press	**60 SECONDS:** Sumo Deadlift High Pull	**60 SECONDS:** Bridge and Press
60 SECONDS: High Knees	**60 SECONDS:** Plank	**60 SECONDS:** Supine Knee Tuck
60 SECONDS: Squat and Press	**60 SECONDS:** Sumo Deadlift High Pull	**60 SECONDS:** Bridge and Press
60 SECONDS: High Knees	**60 SECONDS:** Plank	**60 SECONDS:** Supine Knee Tuck
60 SECONDS: Squat and Press	**60 SECONDS:** Sumo Deadlift High Pull	**60 SECONDS:** Bridge and Press

Week 2

Day 1	Day 2	Day 3
60 SECONDS: Squat and Press with Weight	**60 SECONDS:** Sumo Deadlift High Pull with Weight	**60 SECONDS:** Bridge and Press with Weight
60 SECONDS: Mountain Climbers	**60 SECONDS:** Side Plank	**60 SECONDS:** Cross-Body Mountain Climbers
60 SECONDS: Squat and Press with Weight	**60 SECONDS:** Sumo Deadlift High Pull with Weight	**60 SECONDS:** Bridge and Press with Weight
60 SECONDS: Mountain Climbers	**60 SECONDS:** Side Plank	**60 SECONDS:** Cross-Body Mountain Climbers
60 SECONDS: Squat and Press with Weight	**60 SECONDS:** Sumo Deadlift High Pull with Weight	**60 SECONDS:** Bridge and Press with Weight

Day 4	Day 5	Day 6	Day 7
60 SECONDS: Deadlift and Row	**60 SECONDS:** Burpee	**60 SECONDS:** Overhead Swing	Rest day. Enjoy a family bike ride, walking your dog, or taking a swim.
60 SECONDS: Straight-Arm Plank	**60 SECONDS:** Cross-Body High Knees	**60 SECONDS:** Bird Dog	
60 SECONDS: Deadlift and Row	**60 SECONDS:** Burpee	**60 SECONDS:** Overhead Swing	
60 SECONDS: Straight-Arm Plank	**60 SECONDS:** Cross-Body High Knees	**60 SECONDS:** Bird Dog	
60 SECONDS: Deadlift and Row	**60 SECONDS:** Burpee	**60 SECONDS:** Overhead Swing	

Day 4	Day 5	Day 6	Day 7
60 SECONDS: Deadlift and Row with Weight	**60 SECONDS:** Burpee with Pushup	**60 SECONDS:** Overhead Swing with Weight	Rest day. Try a new sport (even if it's a game of darts) or challenge a friend to a race.
60 SECONDS: Straight-Arm Side Plank	**60 SECONDS:** Bird Dog with Crunch	**60 SECONDS:** Supine Straight-Leg Raise	
60 SECONDS: Deadlift and Row with Weight	**60 SECONDS:** Burpee with Pushup	**60 SECONDS:** Overhead Swing with Weight	
60 SECONDS: Straight-Arm Side Plank	**60 SECONDS:** Bird Dog with Crunch	**60 SECONDS:** Supine Straight-Leg Raise	
60 SECONDS: Deadlift and Row with Weight	**60 SECONDS:** Burpee with Pushup	**60 SECONDS:** Overhead Swing with Weight	

WORKOUT
WEEKS

3-4

AT A
GLANCE

Here you'll
find the
exercises
listed for
each week.
Detailed
descriptions
and photos
for all moves
are in the
next chapter.

Week 3

Day 1	Day 2	Day 3
60 SECONDS: Glider Lunge and Overhead Lift	**60 SECONDS:** Shoulder-Elevated Bridge with Pull-Apart	**60 SECONDS:** Short-Step Backward Lunge with Single-Arm Press
60 SECONDS: Standing Band Pull-Apart	**60 SECONDS:** Around-the-World Elbow Plank	**60 SECONDS:** Resistance Band Press-Out
60 SECONDS: Glider Lunge and Overhead Lift	**60 SECONDS:** Shoulder-Elevated Bridge with Pull-Apart	**60 SECONDS:** Short-Step Backward Lunge with Single-Arm Press
60 SECONDS: Standing Band Pull-Apart	**60 SECONDS:** Around-the-World Elbow Plank	**60 SECONDS:** Resistance Band Press-Out
60 SECONDS: Glider Lunge and Overhead Lift	**60 SECONDS:** Shoulder-Elevated Bridge with Pull-Apart	**60 SECONDS:** Short-Step Backward Lunge with Single-Arm Press

Week 4

Day 1	Day 2	Day 3
60 SECONDS: Goblet Glider Lunge	**60 SECONDS:** Sumo Deadlift with Jump	**60 SECONDS:** Lateral Glider Lunge with Weight
60 SECONDS: High Knees with Overhead Hold	**60 SECONDS:** Leg Lift with Band Stretch	**60 SECONDS:** Torso Twist with Weight
60 SECONDS: Goblet Glider Lunge	**60 SECONDS:** Sumo Deadlift with Jump	**60 SECONDS:** Lateral Glider Lunge with Weight
60 SECONDS: High Knees with Overhead Hold	**60 SECONDS:** Leg Lift with Band Stretch	**60 SECONDS:** Torso Twist with Weight
60 SECONDS: Goblet Glider Lunge	**60 SECONDS:** Sumo Deadlift with Jump	**60 SECONDS:** Lateral Glider Lunge with Weight

Day 4	Day 5	Day 6	Day 7
60 SECONDS: Supine Bridge with Glider	**60 SECONDS:** Long-Step Lunge with Overhead Hold	**60 SECONDS:** Burpee with Overhead Swing	Rest day. Go on a hike, explore a museum, visit family or friends at a park.
60 SECONDS: Around-the-World Elbow Plank	**60 SECONDS:** Cross-Body Wood Chop	**60 SECONDS:** Alternating Leg Lift with Pull-Apart	
60 SECONDS: Supine Bridge with Glider	**60 SECONDS:** Long-Step Lunge with Overhead Hold	**60 SECONDS:** Burpee with Overhead Swing	
60 SECONDS: Around-the-World Elbow Plank	**60 SECONDS:** Cross-Body Wood Chop	**60 SECONDS:** Alternating Leg Lift with Pull-Apart	
60 SECONDS: Supine Bridge with Glider	**60 SECONDS:** Long-Step Lunge with Overhead Hold	**60 SECONDS:** Burpee with Overhead Swing	

Day 4	Day 5	Day 6	Day 7
60 SECONDS: Single-Leg Balance Touch	**60 SECONDS:** Burpee with Weight	**60 SECONDS:** Single-Leg Balance with One-Arm Row	Rest day. Go bird-watching, wash the car outside, or go dancing in or out of the house.
60 SECONDS: Single-Arm Plank	**60 SECONDS:** High Knees with Overhead Hold	**60 SECONDS:** Single-Arm Plank with Rotation	
60 SECONDS: Single-Leg Balance Touch	**60 SECONDS:** Burpee with Weight	**60 SECONDS:** Single-Leg Balance with One-Arm Row	
60 SECONDS: Single-Arm Plank	**60 SECONDS:** High Knees with Overhead Hold	**60 SECONDS:** Single-Arm Plank with Rotation	
60 SECONDS: Single-Leg Balance Touch	**60 SECONDS:** Burpee with Weight	**60 SECONDS:** Single-Leg Balance with One-Arm Row	

"Nothing happens until something starts moving."

—ALBERT EINSTEIN

Here they are—the exercises you'll use to sculpt a brand-new body. To keep the 5-Minute Fitness Formula as simple as possible, I've included instructions and photos for each exercise. It's time to get excited—and get moving!

But first, you need to do something very important. I want you to record some "starting out" stats. This will make it easy for you to track your progress as you go.

1. What is your current weight? _____
2. What is your current waist circumference in inches? _____

Think of this as a little "before" snapshot. Good luck—I know you can do it!

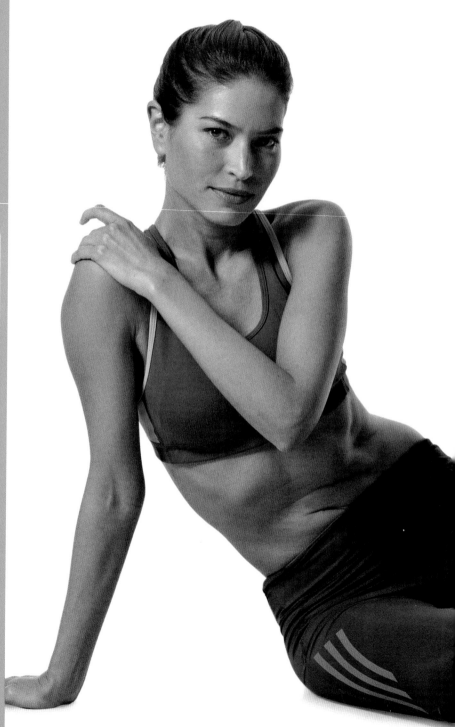

Week
1

Get ready!
It all starts
right here!

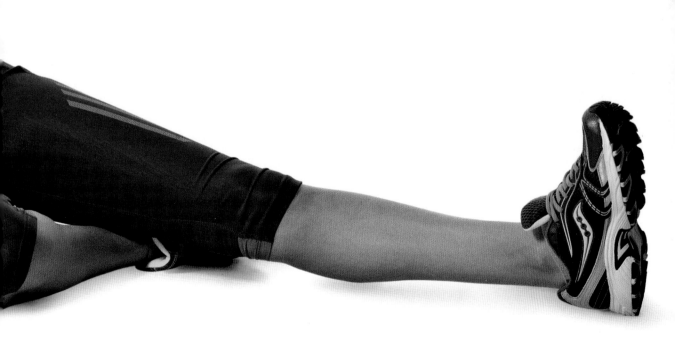

THIS WEEK WILL FOCUS ON
INTRODUCING COMPOUND EXERCISES
INTO YOUR LIFE.
You'll see and feel how these challenging
moves are different from more basic
"single-joint" exercises like a biceps curl.
This week, I want you to use only your body
weight and focus on good form. This is
exciting stuff: You'll be using every muscle
in your body and taking the first steps
to creating a whole new you!

> "The secret of getting ahead is getting started."
>
> —MARK TWAIN

TODAY'S WORKOUT:

60 SECONDS:
Squat and Press

60 SECONDS:
High Knees

60 SECONDS:
Squat and Press

60 SECONDS:
High Knees

60 SECONDS:
Squat and Press

5 minutes and you're done!

SQUAT AND PRESS

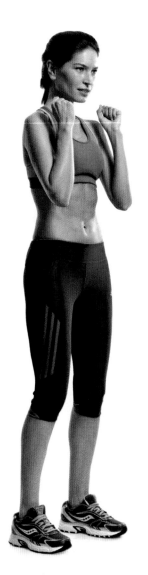

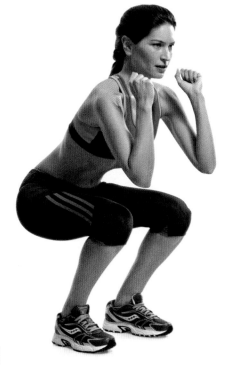

A

Place your feet shoulder-width apart and fists in front of your shoulders.

B

Lower yourself until your hips are at or below your knees. Pause for a second.

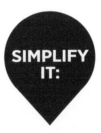

SUPER-CHARGE IT:

As you stand and extend your arms overhead, also lift one knee as high as you can, then lower it as you lower your hands. Alternate knees with each rep.

SIMPLIFY IT:

Squats are most effective if your thighs are parallel to the ground or lower. If you can't do that right now, lower yourself halfway, then complete the rep as described. Your squats will get deeper with time.

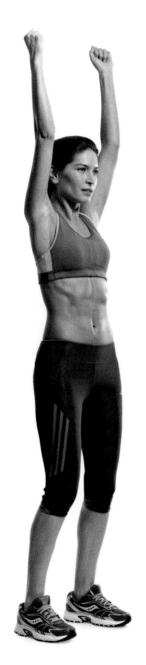

C

Stand up tall while extending your arms overhead. Lower your fists back down. That's 1 rep. Repeat for 60 seconds.

HIGH KNEES

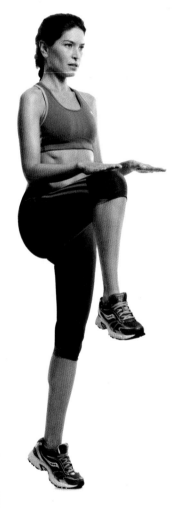

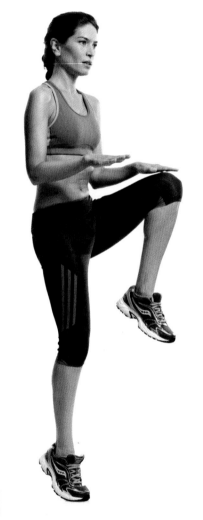

A

Standing tall, place your hands out in front of you with your arms bent at 90 degrees.

B

Lift one knee to the same-side hand and alternate sides for 60 seconds.

"Whether you
think you can
or you can't . . .
you're right."

—HENRY FORD

TODAY'S
WORKOUT:

60 SECONDS:
Sumo Deadlift
High Pull

60 SECONDS:
Plank

60 SECONDS:
Sumo Deadlift
High Pull

60 SECONDS:
Plank

60 SECONDS:
Sumo Deadlift
High Pull

*5 minutes and
you're done!*

SUMO DEADLIFT HIGH PULL

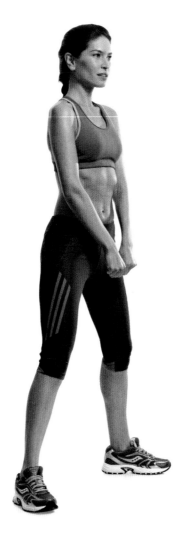

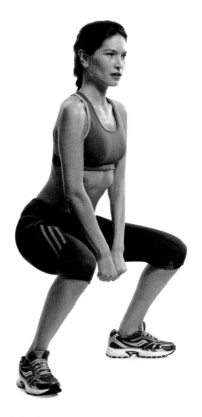

A

Stand with your feet wider than shoulder width and hands in front of your hips, fists touching side by side. Your arms should be straight.

B

Squat while lowering your fists in front of your body until your thighs are parallel to the floor. Pause for a second.

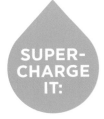

SUPER-CHARGE IT:

After you bring your hands up under your chin, twist your torso to the left while keeping your feet flat on the floor. Pause, then twist to your right. Return to the starting position. This trunk rotation will work your core.

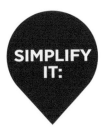

SIMPLIFY IT:

Squats are most effective if your thighs are parallel to the ground or lower. If you can't do that right now, lower yourself halfway, then complete the rep as described. Your squats will get deeper with time.

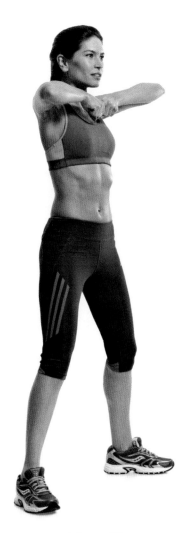

C

Stand up quickly while pulling your fists straight up your torso in front of your chest until you're nearly touching your chin. Lower your arms. That's 1 rep. Repeat for 60 seconds.

PLANK >

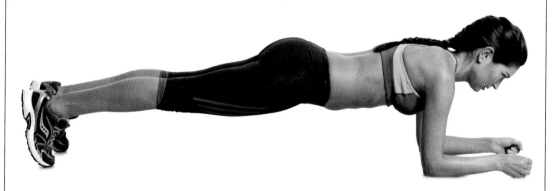

Make like you're going to do a pushup, but rest your weight on your forearms and position your elbows below your shoulders. Your body should form a straight line from your shoulders to your ankles. Brace your core and hold for 60 seconds. (If you can't hold for the entire 60 seconds, take breaks as needed, but try to hold the plank for at least 15 seconds at a stretch. You'll get stronger!)

"Success is dependent upon the glands—the sweat glands."

—ZIG ZIGLAR

TODAY'S WORKOUT:

60 SECONDS:
Bridge and Press

60 SECONDS:
Supine Knee Tuck

60 SECONDS:
Bridge and Press

60 SECONDS:
Supine Knee Tuck

60 SECONDS:
Bridge and Press

5 minutes and you're done!

BRIDGE AND PRESS

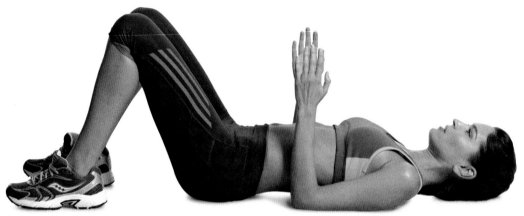

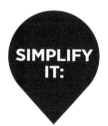

Lie on your back with your feet shoulder-width apart, flat on the ground, and your knees bent at 90 degrees. Bend your elbows 90 degrees so your hands point to the sky.

SIMPLIFY IT: Simply do the bridge part of the exercise without pressing your arms up. As you feel stronger and have more stability, add in the press movement.

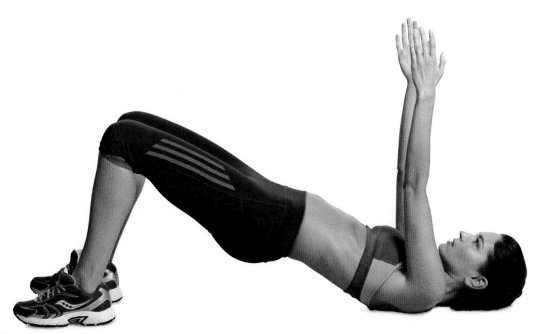

B

Drive your hips up off the ground by squeezing your butt. Lift until your body is a straight line from your knees to your shoulders. At the same time you lift your hips, reach your hands straight up to the sky until your arms are straight.

Hold that position for a 2 count and then lower yourself to the starting position. That's 1 rep. Continue for the entire 60 seconds.

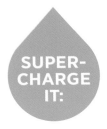

SUPER-CHARGE IT:

At the top of the movement, when your body is straight and your hands are up to the sky, keep your feet flat on the floor but bring your knees together and hold for a 2 count. Then open them and return to the start. This hits the muscles of your inner thighs and outer hips (adductors and abductors).

ANOTHER IDEA: At the top of the movement, keeping your arms straight, open them wide and then lower them to the floor until your hands touch the ground. Hold for a 2 count, then lift your arms back up and return to the start. This gives your chest and shoulders an additional workout.

SUPINE KNEE TUCK

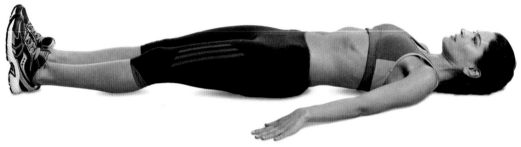

Lie on your back with your legs straight and arms by your sides, palms flat on the floor.

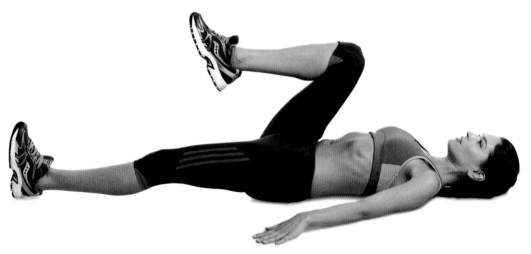

Bend your right knee and lift it up toward your chest. Lift your left knee as you simultaneously lower your right knee in a fluid motion. Alternate knees for the entire 60 seconds.

TODAY'S WORKOUT:

60 SECONDS:
Deadlift and Row

60 SECONDS:
Straight-Arm Plank

60 SECONDS:
Deadlift and Row

60 SECONDS:
Straight-Arm Plank

60 SECONDS:
Deadlift and Row

5 minutes and you're done!

"Nothing great was ever achieved without enthusiasm."

—RALPH WALDO EMERSON

DEADLIFT AND ROW

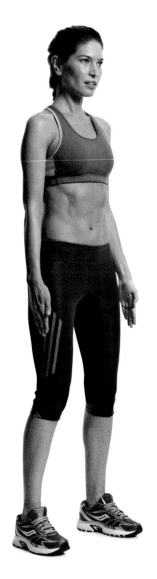

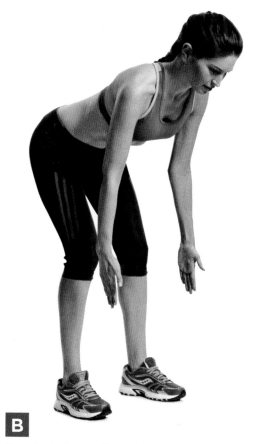

A

Stand tall with your feet as wide as your hips and your hands straight at your sides.

B

Bend at the waist and lower your hands until your torso is parallel with the floor.

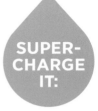

SUPER-CHARGE IT:

In the bottom position, after you do the row and lower your arms, open your arms wide until they're straight out to each side. Squeeze your shoulder blades together as if trying to pinch a coin between them. Hold for a second, then lower and continue the rest of the exercise.

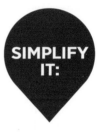

SIMPLIFY IT:

Eliminate the row portion of the exercise, limiting the move to a body-weight deadlift.

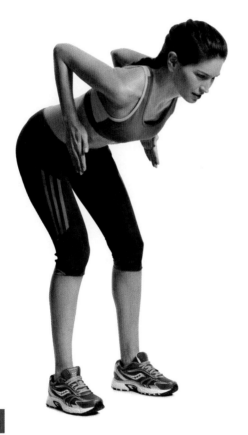

C

While in the bottom position, pull your elbows behind you until your wrists meet your ribs. Hold for a second. Lower your arms, stand up tall, and repeat for 60 seconds.

STRAIGHT-ARM PLANK

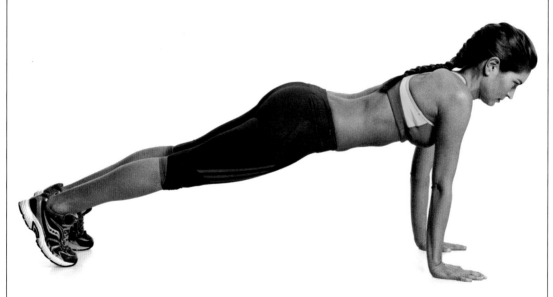

Get into a pushup position, arms straight and your body in a straight line from your shoulders to your feet. Tense your butt and brace your core for 60 seconds. (If you need to, take breaks, but try to hold the plank for at least 15 seconds at a stretch. You'll get stronger!)

WEEK

1 2 3 4

DAY

1 2 3 4 **5** 6

"Perhaps I am stronger than I think."

—THOMAS MERTON

TODAY'S WORKOUT:

60 SECONDS:
Burpee

60 SECONDS:
Cross-Body
High Knees

60 SECONDS:
Burpee

60 SECONDS:
Cross-Body
High Knees

60 SECONDS:
Burpee

*5 minutes and
you're done!*

BURPEE

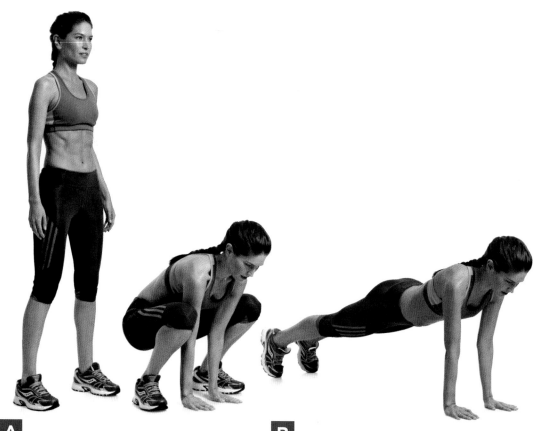

A

Perform the following in quick succession, but in control (proper form is more important than speed).

Stand tall with your feet shoulder-width apart. Squat until your hips are lower than your knees.

B

Place your hands on the floor in between your feet and jump your feet back so you're in a pushup position.

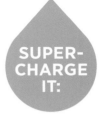

SUPER-CHARGE IT:

Pick one (or do both!): While in a pushup position, do a pushup. Also, when you stand up tall, add in a jump at the end.

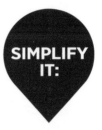

SIMPLIFY IT:

Don't eliminate any portion of the Burpee. Simply go slower. This is a move that will help develop your fast-twitch muscles (the ones that help you do quick, explosive movements). Concentrate on making each movement forceful, but in control. You'll be doing faster reps in no time!

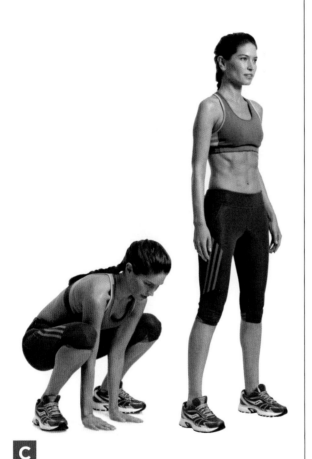

C

Jump your feet back up to your hands and stand up tall, finishing by tensing your butt. Repeat for 60 seconds.

CROSS-BODY HIGH KNEES

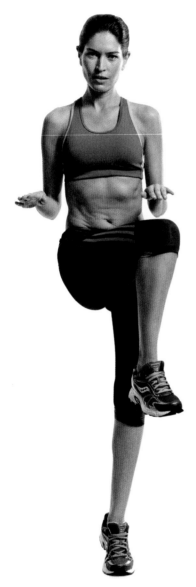 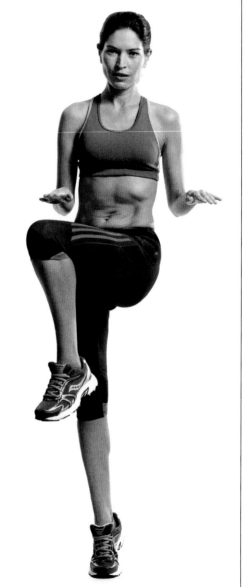

While standing tall with your hands out in front of you and your arms bent at 90 degrees, lift one knee toward your opposite hand. Lower your foot and repeat on the other side, alternating for 60 seconds.

TODAY'S
WORKOUT:

60 SECONDS:
Overhead Swing

60 SECONDS:
Bird Dog

60 SECONDS:
Overhead Swing

60 SECONDS:
Bird Dog

60 SECONDS:
Overhead Swing

*5 minutes and
you're done!*

"The great dividing line between success and failure can be expressed in five words, 'I did not have time.'"

—FRANKLIN FIELD

OVERHEAD SWING

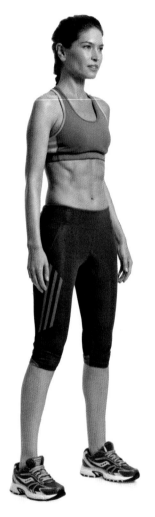

A

Stand with your feet slightly wider than shoulder width.

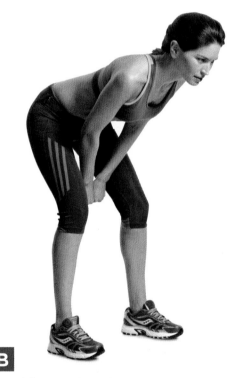

B

Bend forward, slightly bending your knees, and slide your hands in between your legs (keep your fists touching). Hold for a second.

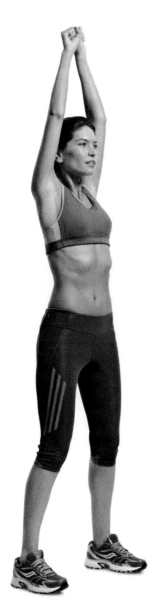

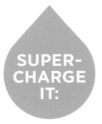

SUPER-CHARGE IT:

At the top of the movement, with your arms straight above your head and your fists touching, spread your arms straight out to either side. Twist to the right, hold for a second, and then twist to the left and hold. Come back to the center and lift arms back up until your fists touch. Continue exercise as described.

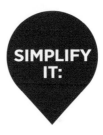

SIMPLIFY IT:

This exercise shouldn't be simplified. It's one of the better total-body moves you can do.

C

Snap your hips forward and stand back up. Let your arms flow overhead while bracing your tummy and squeezing your butt. Hold for a second and then repeat for 60 seconds.

BIRD DOG

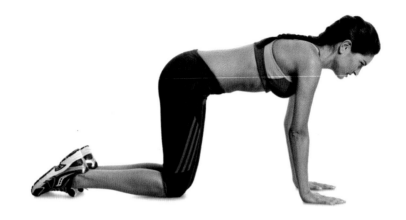

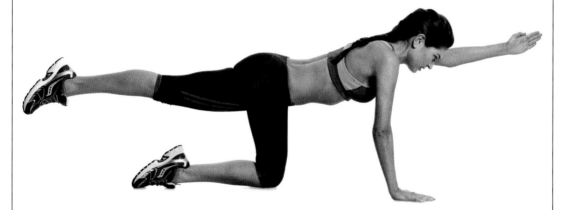

Get on your hands and knees. Lift one arm straight out until it's in line with your ear and extend your opposite leg straight back while clenching your butt. Return your hand and leg to the starting position and repeat on the other side, alternating for 60 seconds.

It's time to monitor your progress! This little exercise will keep you focused and accountable. Just answer the following questions:

1. What is your current weight? Use a scale to weigh yourself and also write down your original weight. _____

2. What have you done well this week? What makes you proud?

_____

_____

_____

3. What could you be doing better? _____

_____

_____

4. What's your game plan for Week 2? _____

_____

_____

One week down—Let's keep moving!

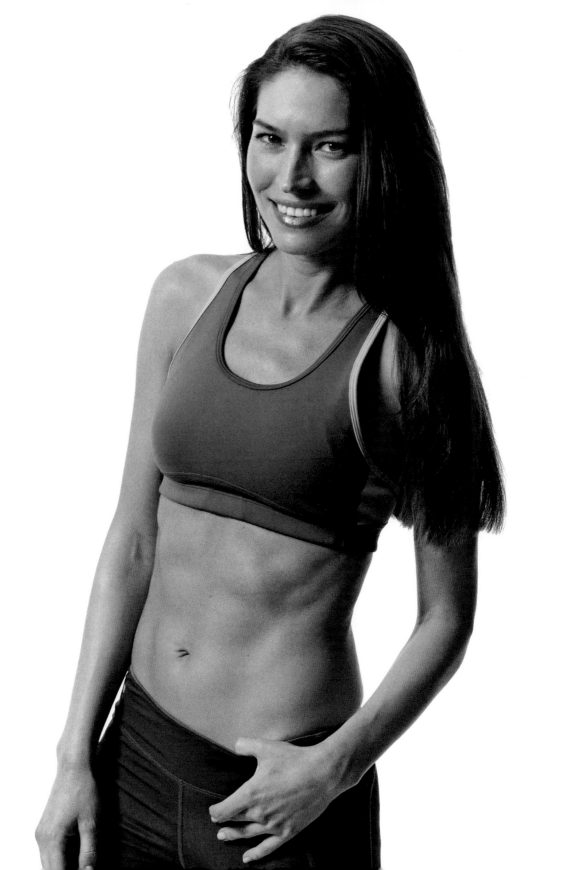

CONGRATULATIONS ON COMPLETING YOUR FIRST WEEK.

By now, you have a very good idea of what compound exercises are, how they feel, and how to approach them. This week, we're going to up the ante. The exercises will still be challenging, and you'll still go 6 days with rest on Sunday. But in some places, we'll add in resistance (that's a fancy word for "weights"). This will help you build more muscle and burn more calories. I want every day to be a stepping-stone to your next day, with you feeling good and moving forward with gains. Five minutes from now, you'll feel even better. Let's go!

"The first wealth is health."

—RALPH WALDO EMERSON

TODAY'S WORKOUT:

60 SECONDS:
Squat and Press
with Weight

60 SECONDS:
Mountain Climbers

60 SECONDS:
Squat and Press
with Weight

60 SECONDS:
Mountain Climbers

60 SECONDS:
Squat and Press
with Weight

*5 minutes and
you're done!*

SQUAT AND PRESS WITH WEIGHT

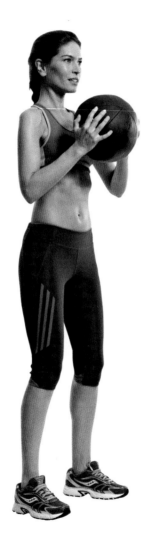

A

While holding a medicine ball (or both ends of a dumbbell) in front of your chest, place your feet shoulder-width apart.

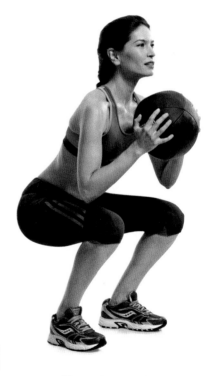

B

Lower yourself until your thighs are parallel to the floor (or squat deeper). Hold for a second.

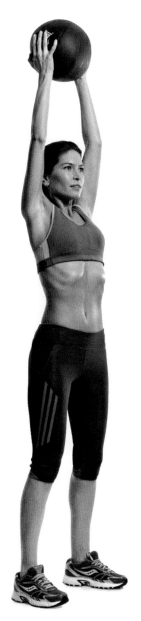

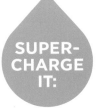

SUPER-CHARGE IT:

As you stand and extend your arms overhead, also lift one knee as high as you can, then lower it as you lower your hands. Alternate knees with each rep.

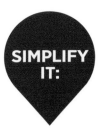

SIMPLIFY IT:

Squats are most effective if your thighs are parallel to the ground or lower. If you can't do that right now, lower yourself halfway, then complete the rep as described. Your squats will get deeper with time.

C

Stand up tall while extending your arms overhead. Lower your hands to your chest. That's 1 rep. Repeat for 60 seconds.

MOUNTAIN CLIMBERS

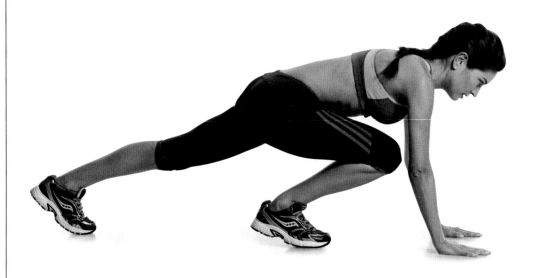

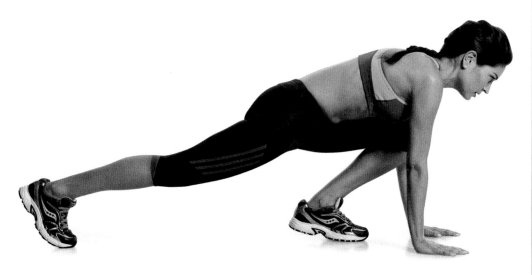

In a pushup position, drive one knee toward the same-side elbow. Return your foot to the starting position and repeat with the other leg as fast as possible for 60 seconds.

TODAY'S WORKOUT:

60 SECONDS:
Sumo Deadlift
High Pull
with Weight

60 SECONDS:
Side Plank

60 SECONDS:
Sumo Deadlift
High Pull
with Weight

60 SECONDS:
Side Plank

60 SECONDS:
Sumo Deadlift
High Pull
with Weight

*5 minutes and
you're done!*

"It's never too late to be what you might have been."

—GEORGE ELIOT

SUMO DEADLIFT HIGH PULL WITH WEIGHT

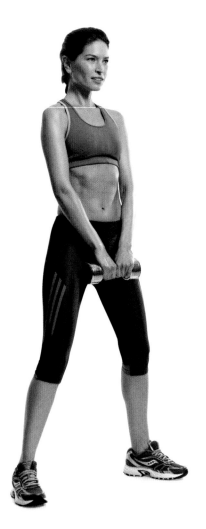

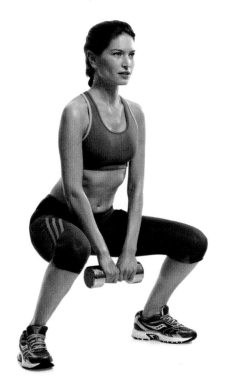

A

Stand with your feet wider than shoulder width and hands in front of your hips, holding a dumbbell (or medicine ball). Your arms should be straight.

B

Squat while lowering your hands in front of your body until your thighs are parallel to the floor. Pause for a second.

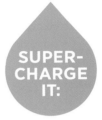

SUPER-CHARGE IT:

After you bring your hands up under your chin, twist your torso to the left while keeping your feet flat on the floor. Pause, then twist to your right. Return to the starting position. This trunk rotation will work your core.

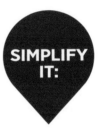

SIMPLIFY IT:

Squats are most effective if your thighs are parallel to the ground or lower. If you can't do that right now, lower yourself halfway, then complete the rep as described. Your squats will get deeper with time.

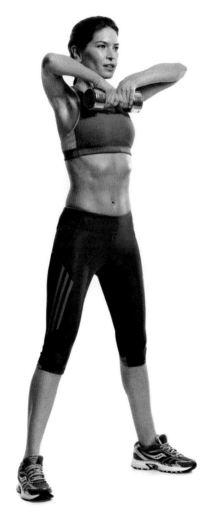

C

Stand up quickly while lifting the weight straight up your torso in front of your chest until you're nearly touching your chin. Lower your arms. That's 1 rep. Repeat for 60 seconds.

SIDE PLANK

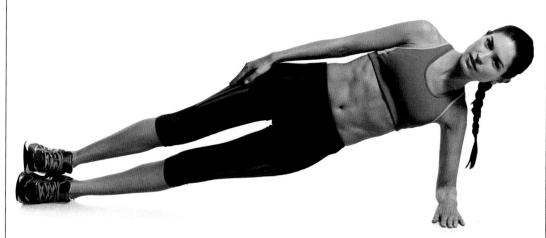

Lie on your side with your feet stacked on top of one another and your elbow aligned under your shoulder. Elevate your butt off the ground so your body is in a straight line from your head to your ankles. Hold for 30 seconds. Switch to the other side and hold for 30 seconds.

TODAY'S
WORKOUT:

60 SECONDS:
Bridge and Press
with Weight

60 SECONDS:
Cross-Body
Mountain Climbers

60 SECONDS:
Bridge and Press
with Weight

60 SECONDS:
Cross-Body
Mountain Climbers

60 SECONDS:
Bridge and Press
with Weight

*5 minutes and
you're done!*

"Go out on a limb. That's where the fruit is."

—WILL ROGERS

BRIDGE AND PRESS WITH WEIGHT

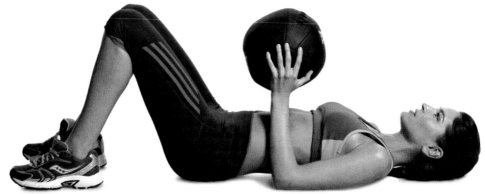

A

While holding a medicine ball (or both ends of a dumbbell) in your hands close to your chest, lie on your back with your feet shoulder-width apart, flat on the ground, and your knees bent at 90 degrees.

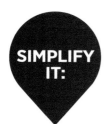

SIMPLIFY IT: Simply do the bridge part of the exercise without pressing your arms up. As you feel stronger and have more stability, add in the press movement.

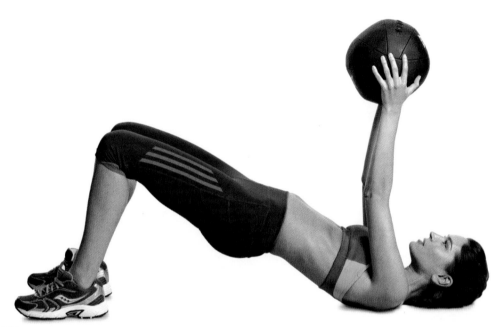

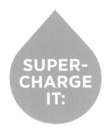

Drive your hips up off the ground by squeezing your butt. Lift until your body is a straight line from your knees to your shoulders. At the same time you lift your hips, in a fluid movement, lift the weight up to the sky until your arms are straight.

Hold that position for a 2 count and then lower yourself to the starting position. That's 1 rep. Continue for the entire 60 seconds.

SUPER-CHARGE IT:
At the top of the movement, when your body is straight and your hands are up to the sky, keep your feet flat on the floor but bring your knees together and hold for a 2 count. Then open them and return to the start. This hits the muscles of your inner thighs and outer hips (adductors and abductors).

ANOTHER IDEA: At the top of the movement, when the weight is pressed above you and your arms are straight, lower the weight back behind your head until it touches the floor (your arms remain straight through the movement and end up next to your ears at this point). Hold for a second and lift the weight back up above you.

CROSS-BODY MOUNTAIN CLIMBERS

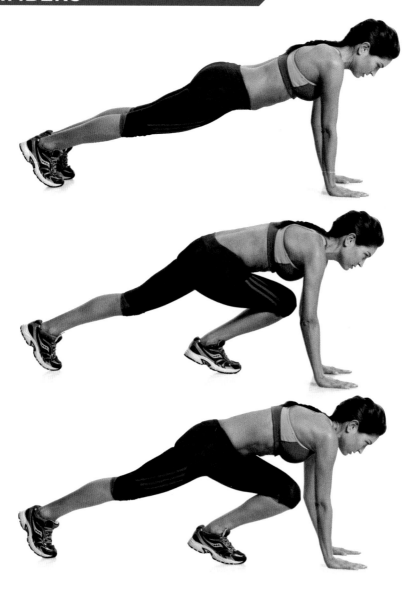

In a pushup position, drive one knee toward the opposite elbow. Return your foot to the starting position and repeat with the other leg as fast as possible for 60 seconds.

TODAY'S WORKOUT:

60 SECONDS:
Deadlift and Row
with Weight

60 SECONDS:
Straight-Arm
Side Plank

60 SECONDS:
Deadlift and Row
with Weight

60 SECONDS:
Straight-Arm
Side Plank

60 SECONDS:
Deadlift and Row
with Weight

*5 minutes and
you're done!*

"There are no shortcuts to any place worth going."

—UNKNOWN

DEADLIFT AND ROW WITH WEIGHT

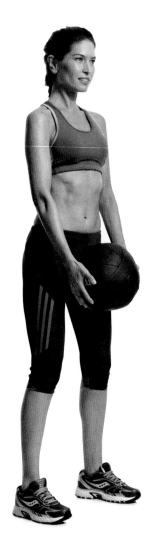

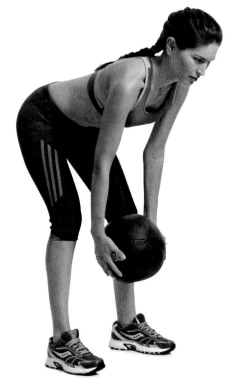

A

Stand tall with your feet as wide as your hips. While holding a medicine ball (or both ends of a dumbbell) in front of your hips, bend at the waist.

B

As you bend, lower the weight down your legs until your torso is parallel with the floor.

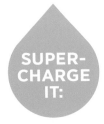

SUPER-CHARGE IT:

As you finish the exercise, add an overhead press to the move by lifting the weight over your head until your arms are straight. Hold for a second, and then lower to the starting position.

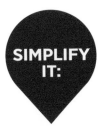

SIMPLIFY IT:

Eliminate the row portion of the exercise, limiting the move to a body-weight deadlift.

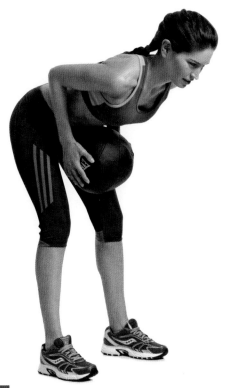

C

While in the bottom position, pull your elbows behind you until the weight meets your ribs. Hold for a second. Lower your arms, stand up tall, and repeat for 60 seconds.

STRAIGHT-ARM SIDE PLANK

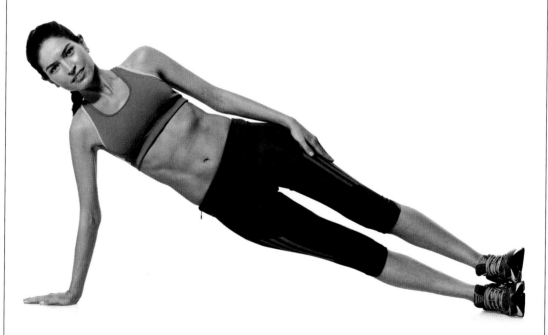

Get into a pushup position. Lift your left arm and turn your torso so your right arm supports your body and your left arm is against your side. Keep your body in a straight line from your head to your ankles and hold for 30 seconds. Switch to the other side and hold for 30 seconds.

TODAY'S WORKOUT:

60 SECONDS:
Burpee with
Pushup

60 SECONDS:
Bird Dog
with Crunch

60 SECONDS:
Burpee with
Pushup

60 SECONDS:
Bird Dog
with Crunch

60 SECONDS:
Burpee with
Pushup

*5 minutes and
you're done!*

"Doing the best at this moment puts you in the best place for the next moment."

—OPRAH WINFREY

BURPEE WITH PUSHUP

Perform the following in quick succession, but in control (proper form is more important than speed).

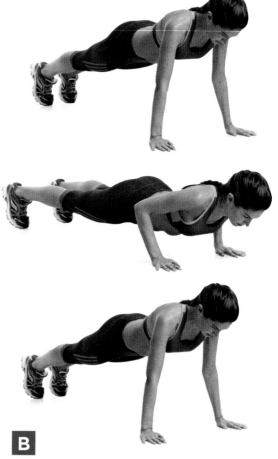
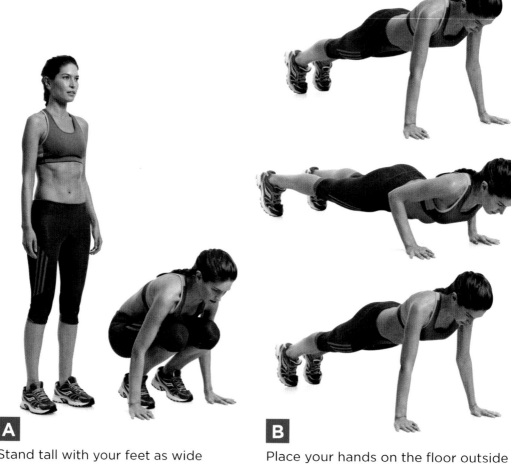

A

Stand tall with your feet as wide as your hips. Squat until your hips are lower than your knees.

B

Place your hands on the floor outside your feet and jump your feet back so you're in a pushup position.

Do a pushup.

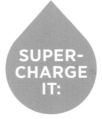

SUPER-CHARGE IT:

Pick one (or do both!): While in a pushup position, do an extra pushup. Also, when you stand up tall, add in a jump at the end.

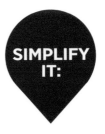

SIMPLIFY IT:

Don't eliminate any portion of the Burpee. Simply go slower. This is a move that will help develop your fast-twitch muscles (the ones that help you do quick, explosive movements). Concentrate on making each movement forceful, but in control. You'll be doing faster reps in no time!

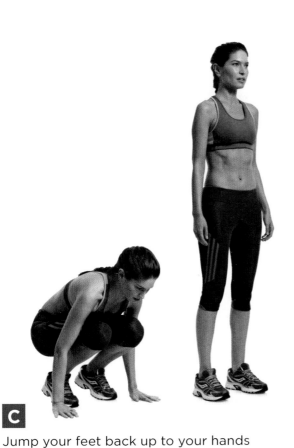

C

Jump your feet back up to your hands and stand up tall, finishing by tensing your butt. Repeat for 60 seconds.

BIRD DOG WITH CRUNCH

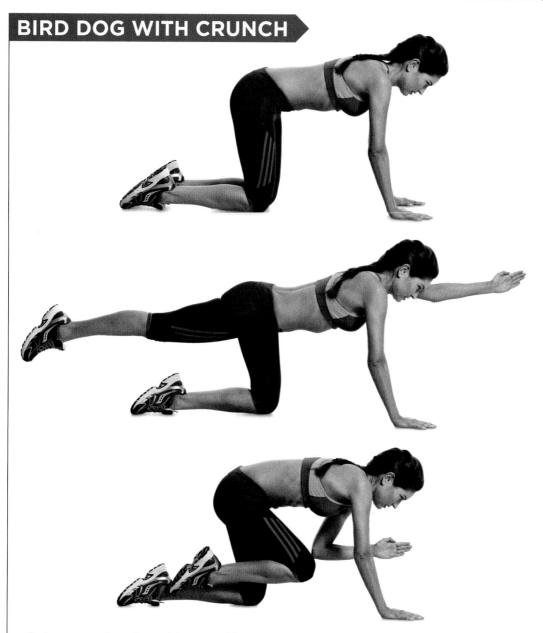

Get on your hands and knees. Lift one arm straight out until your arm is in line with your ear and extend your opposite leg straight back while tensing your butt. Bring your extended arm and leg into your body and touch your elbow and knee, feeling the contraction in your core. Return to the start. That's 1 rep. Repeat for 30 seconds, then switch to the other side for 30 seconds.

TODAY'S WORKOUT:

60 SECONDS:
Overhead Swing with Weight

60 SECONDS:
Supine Straight-Leg Raise

60 SECONDS:
Overhead Swing with Weight

60 SECONDS:
Supine Straight-Leg Raise

60 SECONDS:
Overhead Swing with Weight

5 minutes and you're done!

"Practice puts brains in your muscles."

—SAM SNEAD

OVERHEAD SWING WITH WEIGHT

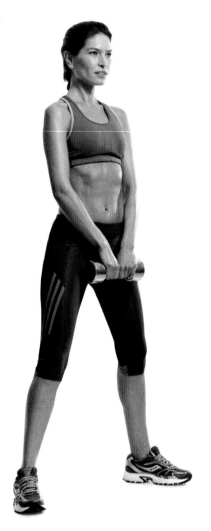

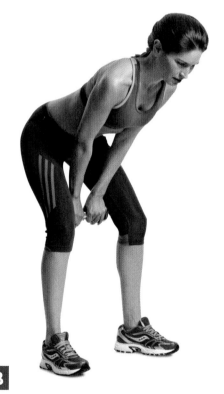

A

Stand with your feet slightly wider than shoulder width. Let your arms hang in front of you holding a dumbbell (or a medicine ball).

B

As you bend forward, slightly bending your knees, slide your hands between your legs. Hold for a second.

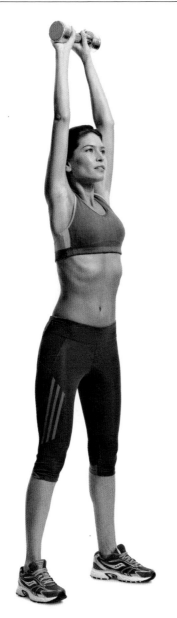

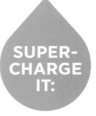

SUPER-CHARGE IT:

At the top of the movement, with the weight straight above your head, lean your torso to the right while keeping your arms straight. Return to the center and lean to the left. Continue the exercise as described.

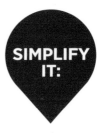

SIMPLIFY IT:

This exercise shouldn't be simplified. It's one of the better total-body moves you can do.

C

Snap your hips forward and stand back up. Let your arms flow overhead with the weight while bracing your tummy and squeezing your butt. Hold for a second and then repeat for 60 seconds.

SUPINE STRAIGHT-LEG RAISE

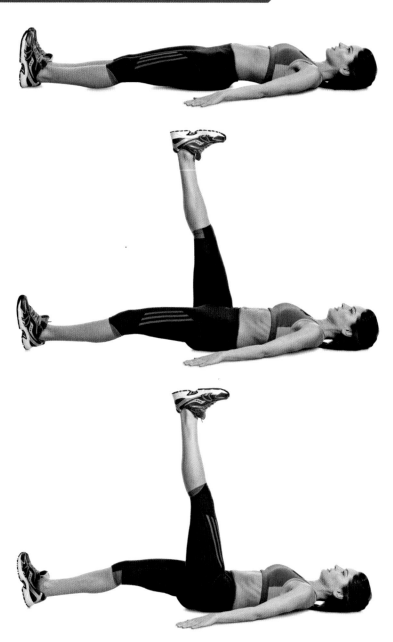

While lying on your back with your arms and legs straight, lift one leg up and down and then repeat with the other leg. Continue for the entire 60 seconds.

It's time to monitor your progress! This little exercise will keep you focused and accountable. Just answer the following questions:

1. What is your current weight? Use a scale to weigh yourself and also write down your original weight. _____

2. What have you done well this week? What makes you proud?

_____
_____
_____

3. What could you be doing better? _____

_____
_____

4. What's your game plan for Week 3? _____

_____
_____

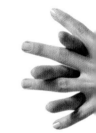

Week
3

14 days
down!
14 more
to go!

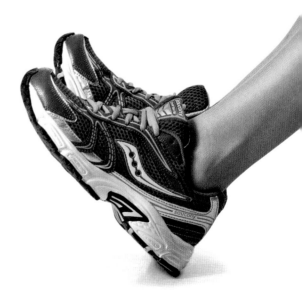

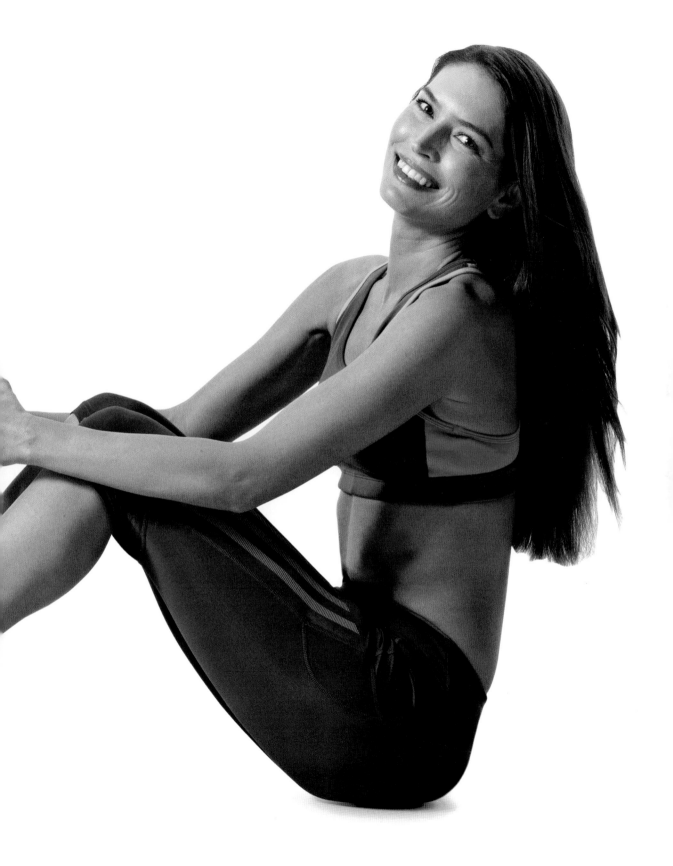

I HOPE YOU FEEL AS GOOD ABOUT REACHING THE HALFWAY POINT OF THE INCHES OFF! PLAN AS I DO JUST THINKING ABOUT IT.

By now, you should be feeling stronger and lighter in your step and have more energy each day. In Week 3, we're going to make the exercises more interesting, adding more resistance and taking advantage of your more powerful body. We really want to build on your previous success and take you to another level this week. So get ready, turn the page, and imagine how much better you'll feel 5 minutes from now!

TODAY'S WORKOUT:

60 SECONDS:
Glider Lunge and Overhead Lift

60 SECONDS:
Standing Band Pull-Apart

60 SECONDS:
Glider Lunge and Overhead Lift

60 SECONDS:
Standing Band Pull-Apart

60 SECONDS:
Glider Lunge and Overhead Lift

5 minutes and you're done!

"The past doesn't define you. Your present does."

—JILLIAN MICHAELS

GLIDER LUNGE AND OVERHEAD LIFT

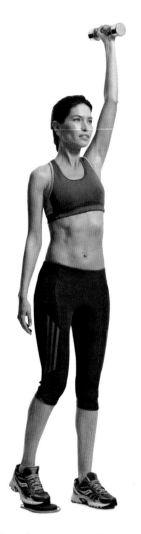

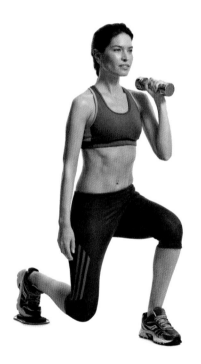

A

Stand with your right foot on a glider or paper plate and a dumbbell in your left hand. Start with the weight held up over your head, arm straight.

B

Slide your gliding foot back until your back knee almost touches the ground. As you move back, lower the weight to shoulder level. Hold for a second.

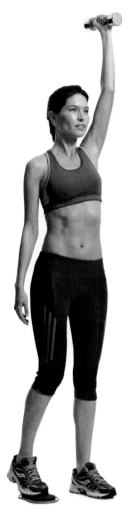

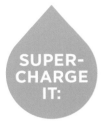

SUPER-CHARGE IT:

If you hold the weight in your left hand, add in a torso twist to the right as you go through the movement so you're facing to the right at the bottom. Return to face front as you return to the starting position. Switch your twist to the left when you switch sides after 30 seconds.

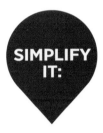

SIMPLIFY IT:

If you can't go all the way back until your knee almost touches the ground, go back halfway. Still, make sure you do the entire dumbbell lift throughout the movement.

C

Glide your foot back up to the standing position while simultaneously lifting the weight straight up in front of you as you stand tall. That's 1 rep.

Repeat for 30 seconds and switch to the other leg and arm for 30 seconds.

STANDING BAND PULL-APART

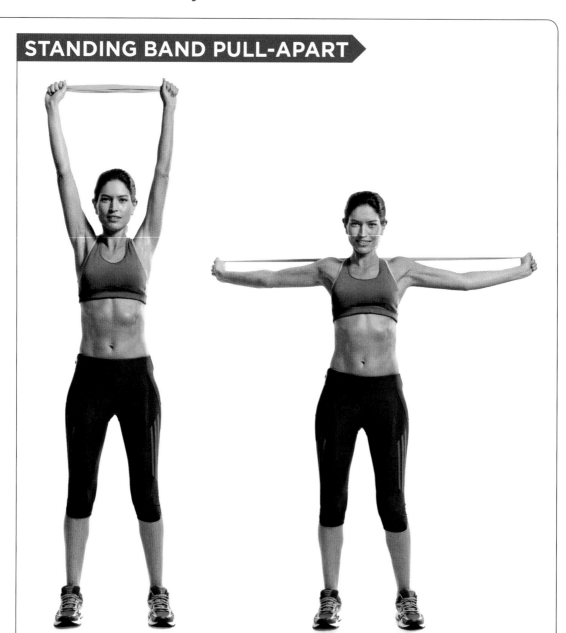

In a standing position, hold a resistance band shoulder-width apart over your head with your arms straight. Tense your butt and brace your abs as you pull outward with both hands until the band touches behind your neck and your arms are straight out at your sides. Squeeze your shoulder blades together during the move. Hold for a second and slowly return to the starting position. That's 1 rep. Repeat for 60 seconds.

TODAY'S WORKOUT:

60 SECONDS:
Shoulder-Elevated
Bridge with
Pull-Apart

60 SECONDS:
Around-the-World
Elbow Plank

60 SECONDS:
Shoulder-Elevated
Bridge with
Pull-Apart

60 SECONDS:
Around-the-World
Elbow Plank

60 SECONDS:
Shoulder-Elevated
Bridge with
Pull-Apart

*5 minutes and
you're done!*

"Happiness is when what you think, what you say, and what you do are in harmony."

—MAHATMA GANDHI

SHOULDER-ELEVATED BRIDGE WITH PULL-APART

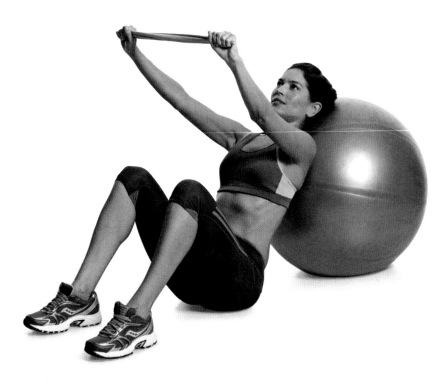

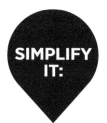

A

To start, grab a resistance band and position your neck and shoulders on a stability ball or bench so you have support. Plant your feet flat on the ground, bend your knees 90 degrees, and lower your butt to the floor. You're in the starting position.

SIMPLIFY IT: Try the exercise without the resistance band, using only your arms. Add it back in when you feel stronger.

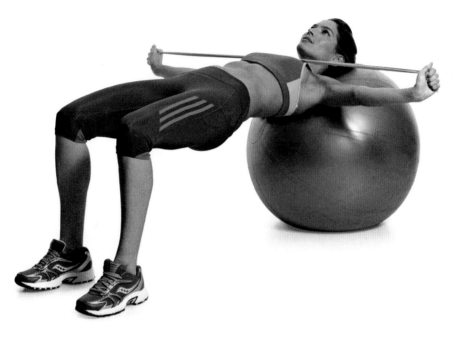

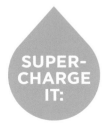

B

Hold the resistance band shoulder-width apart over your chest with your arms straight up in the air. Simultaneously drive your hips up off the ground and pull the band apart until your arms are open wide and the band hits your chest. Your torso should be in a straight line from your head to your knees. Return to the starting position and repeat for 60 seconds.

SUPER-CHARGE IT:

Once your body is straight and the resistance band pulled tight, lift your right foot until your leg is straight. Hold for a second. Lower it and complete the exercise as described. Alternate legs on each rep.

AROUND-THE-WORLD ELBOW PLANK

Lie on your side with your feet stacked on top of one another and shoulder over your elbow. Rotate your chest toward the floor so that both elbows are on the ground and continue until your opposite elbow and foot are on the ground. Continue to roll from one side to the other for 60 seconds.

TODAY'S
WORKOUT:

60 SECONDS:
Short-Step Back-
ward Lunge with
Single-Arm Press

60 SECONDS:
Resistance Band
Press-Out

60 SECONDS:
Short-Step Back-
ward Lunge with
Single-Arm Press

60 SECONDS:
Resistance Band
Press-Out

60 SECONDS:
Short-Step Back-
ward Lunge with
Single-Arm Press

*5 minutes and
you're done!*

"If you do what you've always done, you'll always get what you've always gotten."

—TONY ROBBINS

SHORT-STEP BACKWARD LUNGE WITH SINGLE-ARM PRESS

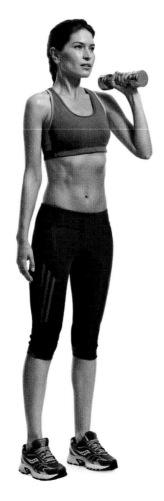

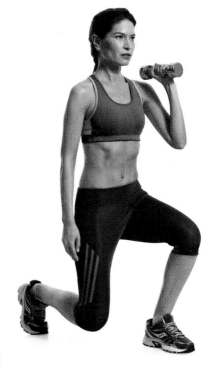

A

Stand with your feet close together and hold a dumbbell in your right hand at shoulder height.

B

Take a small step back with your right leg and lower your body until your right knee almost touches the ground.

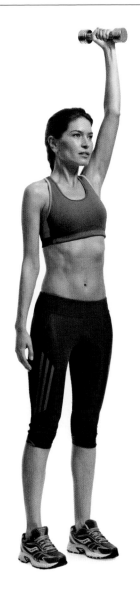

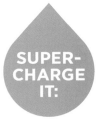

SUPER-CHARGE IT:

Add in a torso twist to the right as you lower, returning to face forward as you rise. When you switch the dumbbell to your left hand after 30 seconds, twist to the left for the next 30 seconds.

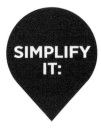

SIMPLIFY IT:

Try it without the dumbbell. Add weight as you get stronger.

C

Stand back up while pressing the weight overhead. That's 1 rep. For subsequent reps, lower the weight as you lower your body and lift the weight as you stand up. Perform for 30 seconds, then switch the dumbbell to your other hand and lunge on your other leg for 30 seconds.

RESISTANCE BAND PRESS-OUT

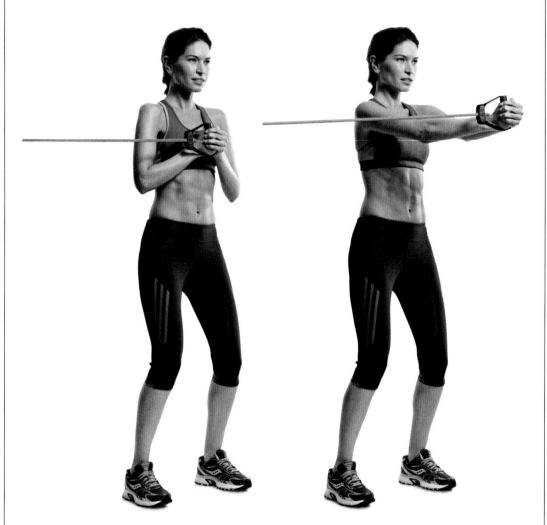

Attach a resistance band to a secure object at chest height (if you're not in a gym, a stair railing, basement pole, or playground equipment works well). Stand to the left of the object, pulling the band until it's taut. Hold it with both hands close to your chest. Brace your core, and without allowing the band to pull your hands to the right, press your hands out straight. Hold for a second, and then return to the starting position. Perform reps for 30 seconds, then switch so the band is attached to your left and repeat for 30 seconds.

**TODAY'S
WORKOUT:**

60 SECONDS:
Supine Bridge
with Glider

60 SECONDS:
Around-the-World
Elbow Plank

60 SECONDS:
Supine Bridge
with Glider

60 SECONDS:
Around-the-World
Elbow Plank

60 SECONDS:
Supine Bridge
with Glider

*5 minutes and
you're done!*

"You gotta
have a body."
—JAYNE MANSFIELD

SUPINE BRIDGE WITH GLIDER

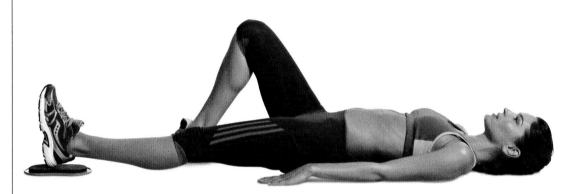

Lie on your back with your arms at your sides, legs flat. Place a glider under your left heel. Raise your right leg so your knee is bent and your right foot is flat on the floor. This is the starting position.

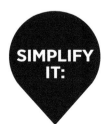

SIMPLIFY IT: This exercise shouldn't be simplified. It's a great way to hit muscles almost literally from head to toe!

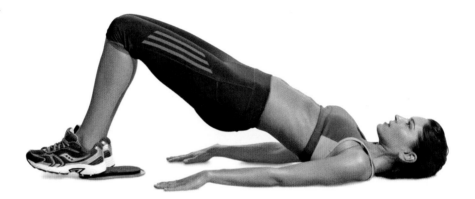

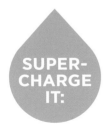

B

Simultaneously lift your butt up and slide your glider leg in toward your body until your feet are next to each other and your torso is in a straight line from your neck to your knees. Hold for a second.

Lower your butt and slide your glider foot out flat. That's 1 rep. Perform on this side for 30 seconds and then switch legs and repeat for 30 seconds.

SUPER-CHARGE IT:

When you reach the top of the movement, spread your knees wide. Hold for a second. Bring them together and finish the exercise as described.

AROUND-THE-WORLD ELBOW PLANK

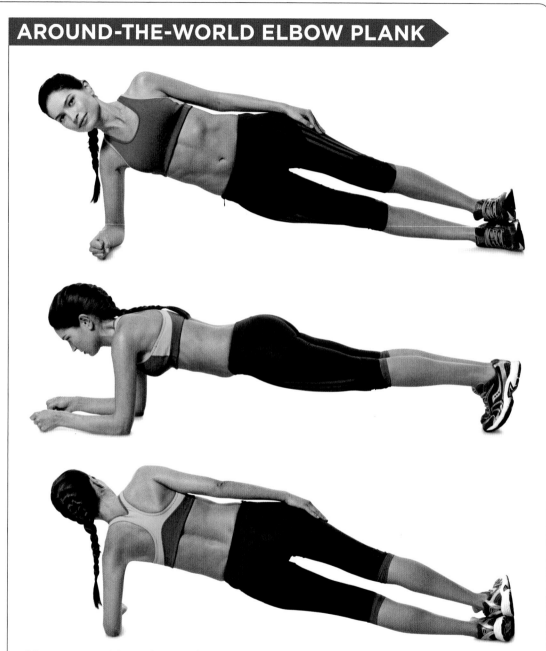

Lie on your side with your feet stacked on top of one another and shoulder over your elbow. Rotate your chest toward the floor so that both elbows are on the ground and continue until your opposite elbow and foot are on the ground. Continue to roll from one side to the other for 60 seconds.

TODAY'S WORKOUT:

60 SECONDS:
Long-Step Lunge with Overhead Hold

60 SECONDS:
Cross-Body Wood Chop

60 SECONDS:
Long-Step Lunge with Overhead Hold

60 SECONDS:
Cross-Body Wood Chop

60 SECONDS:
Long-Step Lunge with Overhead Hold

5 minutes and you're done!

"There's no dream that's too big."
—LADY GAGA

LONG-STEP LUNGE WITH OVERHEAD HOLD

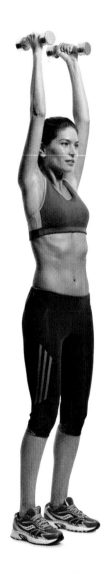

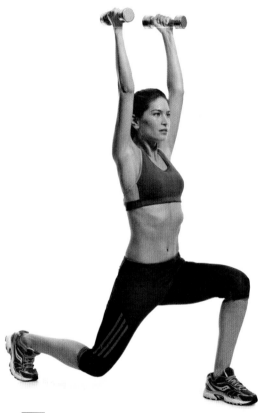

A

Grab a pair of dumbbells and stand with your arms overhead, elbows stiff.

B

Without lowering the dumbbells, take a long step back with your right leg until your right knee almost touches the ground. Return to the standing position.

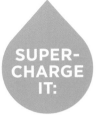

SUPER-CHARGE IT:

When your right leg goes back, add in a torso twist to the left. Return to facing forward as you stand. When you switch to your left leg after 30 seconds, twist to the right.

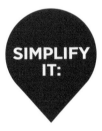

SIMPLIFY IT:

Try it without the dumbbells while still keeping your hands overhead. Add in weight as you get stronger.

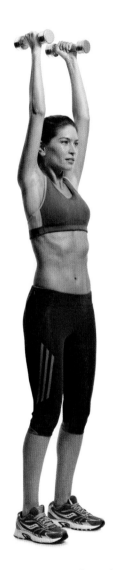

Keep the weights overhead the entire time. Continue for 30 seconds and repeat with the left leg.

CROSS-BODY WOOD CHOP

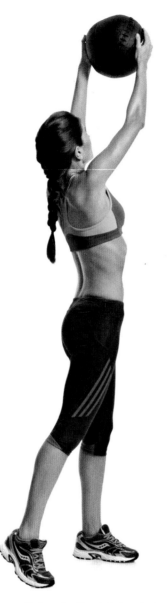
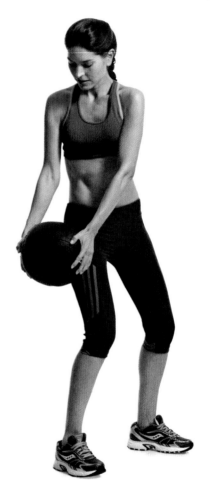

Hold a medicine ball with both hands. Raise the ball up over your left shoulder (as if you want to throw it). Without letting go, swing the ball down across your body until the ball is by your right hip. Repeat the movement for 30 seconds, and then switch to your right shoulder/left hip for 30 seconds.

TODAY'S
WORKOUT:

60 SECONDS:
Burpee with
Overhead Swing

60 SECONDS:
Alternating Leg Lift
with Pull-Apart

60 SECONDS:
Burpee with
Overhead Swing

60 SECONDS:
Alternating Leg Lift
with Pull-Apart

60 SECONDS:
Burpee with
Overhead Swing

*5 minutes and
you're done!*

"With the new day comes new strength and new thoughts."
—ELEANOR ROOSEVELT

BURPEE WITH OVERHEAD SWING

Perform the following in quick succession, but in control (proper form is more important than speed).

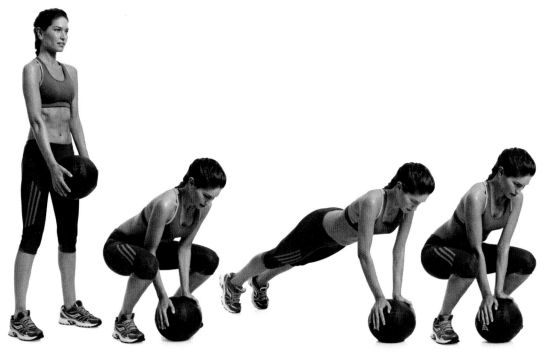

A

Stand with a medicine ball in your hands (you can also use two hexagonal dumbbells). Squat while lowering the medicine ball between your legs until it's on the ground.

B

Jump your feet back so you're in a pushup position (with the ball acting as the base for your hands). Immediately jump your feet back into a squatting position and then stand.

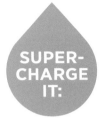

SUPER-CHARGE IT:

When you get into a pushup position, do a pushup (or two!).

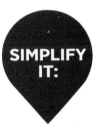

SIMPLIFY IT:

Try the exercise without weight, swinging your hands as described. Add in weight as you get stronger.

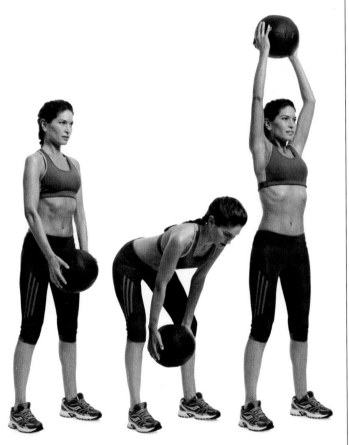

C

Swing the ball back between your legs while bending at the waist and knees. Snap your hips forward and swing the ball up until it's straight up above you.

Lower it and return to the starting position. Repeat for 60 seconds.

ALTERNATING LEG LIFT WITH PULL-APART

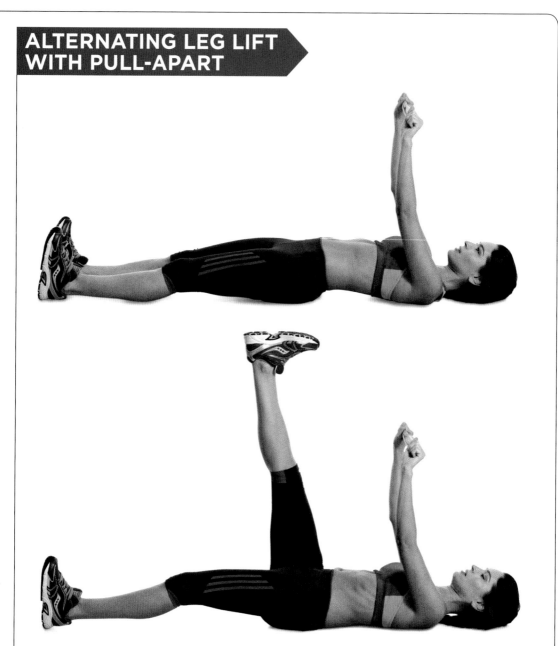

Lie on your back with your legs straight. Hold a resistance band with your hands shoulder-width apart and raised straight above you. Simultaneously lift one leg until it's straight up (don't bend your knee!) while pulling the resistance band apart by opening your arms wide. Lower the leg and return hands to the starting position. Repeat for 60 seconds, alternating legs.

It's time to monitor your progress! This little exercise will keep you focused and accountable. Just answer the following questions:

1. What is your current weight? Use a scale to weigh yourself and also write down your original weight. _____

2. What have you done well this week? What makes you proud?

_____

_____

_____

3. What could you be doing better? _____

_____

_____

4. What's your game plan for Week 4? _____

_____

_____

Week

4

Three
weeks
down—
one week
to go!
Let's raise
the bar!

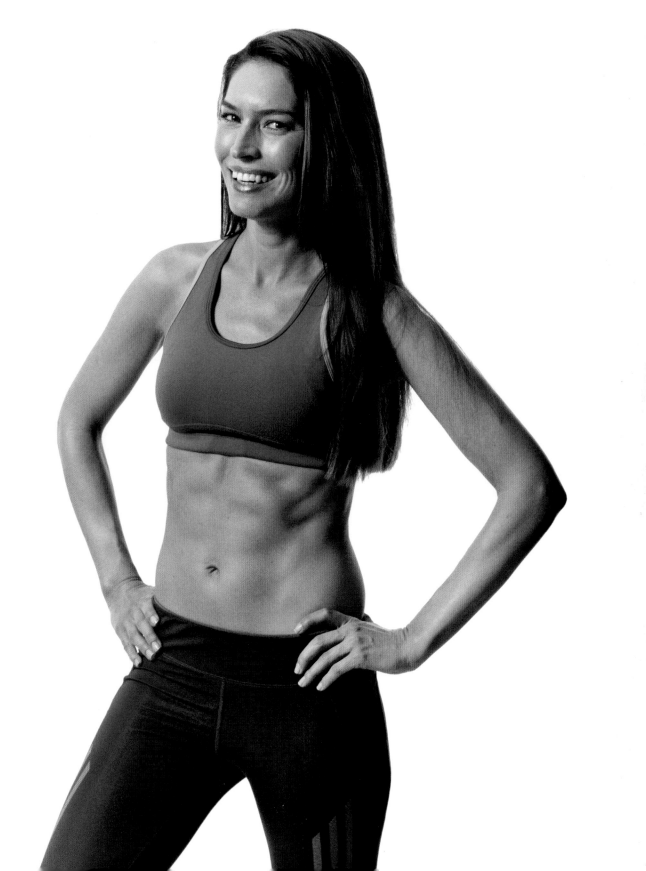

I KNOW YOU'RE SMILING AS YOU READ "ONE WEEK TO GO,"

but I hope you smile not because you're almost done with the Inches Off! 4-week plan, but because you're excited to keep going. You've accomplished so much, and you should be proud of yourself. Now prepare for the final push. This week we'll give you the most challenging exercises yet, adding more weight and encouraging you to push harder to fit even more reps into your 5 minutes. That's the beauty of compound exercises: The harder you work, the more total-body movement you fit into a small amount of time. You've had time to harness real gains and understand how these exercises work. Now's the time to turn yourself loose and really work it. Let's turn the page and have some fun!

TODAY'S WORKOUT:

60 SECONDS:
Goblet Glider Lunge

60 SECONDS:
High Knees with Overhead Hold

60 SECONDS:
Goblet Glider Lunge

60 SECONDS:
High Knees with Overhead Hold

60 SECONDS:
Goblet Glider Lunge

5 minutes and you're done!

"Small deeds done are better than great deeds planned."

—PETER MARSHALL

GOBLET GLIDER LUNGE

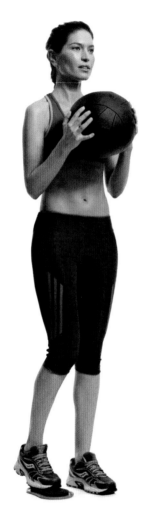

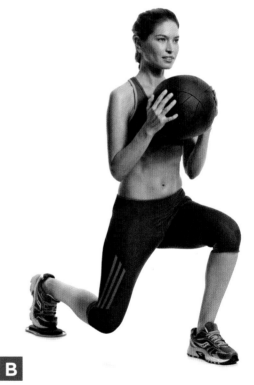

A

Stand tall holding a medicine ball (or two dumbbells) in front of your shoulders and chest. Put a glider or paper plate under your right foot.

B

Slide the glider back until your knee almost touches the ground.

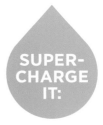

SUPER-CHARGE IT:

As you lower to the floor, add in a torso twist. As you rise, return to facing forward. For your right glider foot, twist left. For the left glider foot, twist right.

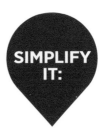

SIMPLIFY IT:

Try it without weight, but hopefully this exercise doesn't have to be simplified. It's a great way to work a huge number of muscles throughout your body.

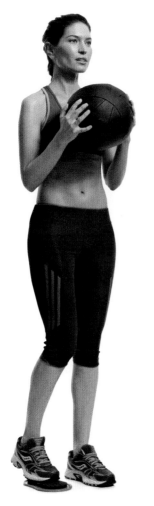

C

Return to a standing position. Repeat for 30 seconds and then switch to your left foot and work the other side for 30 seconds.

HIGH KNEES WITH OVERHEAD HOLD

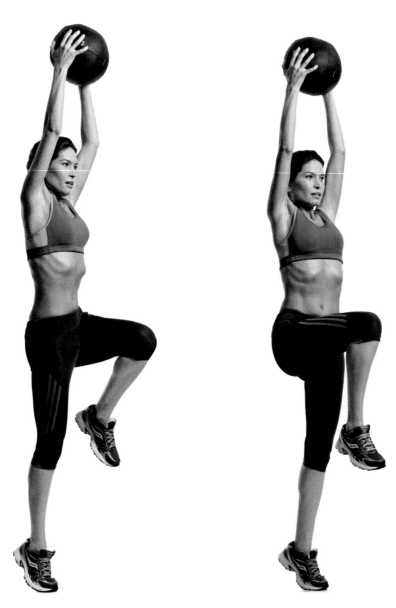

Stand while holding a medicine ball or two dumbbells overhead. While holding the weight up, drive one knee up until it's parallel with your hips. Repeat by alternating legs for 60 seconds. Don't lower the weight until you're finished.

TODAY'S WORKOUT:

60 SECONDS:
Sumo Deadlift
with Jump

60 SECONDS:
Leg Lift
with Band Stretch

60 SECONDS:
Sumo Deadlift
with Jump

60 SECONDS:
Leg Lift
with Band Stretch

60 SECONDS:
Sumo Deadlift
with Jump

5 minutes and you're done!

"A dream doesn't become a reality through magic. It takes sweat, determination, and hard work."

—COLIN POWELL

SUMO DEADLIFT WITH JUMP

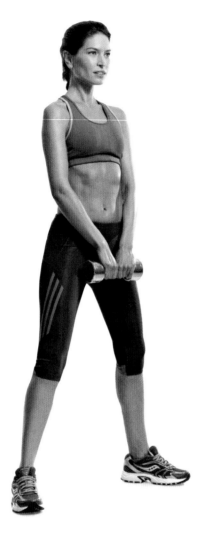

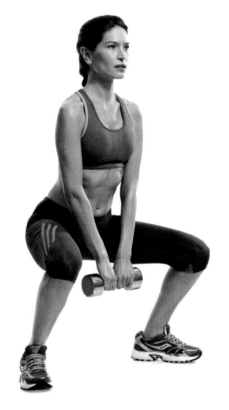

A

Stand with your feet wider than shoulder width and hold a dumbbell (or medicine ball) in your hands, arms straight down in front of you.

B

Squat until your thighs are parallel to the floor. The weight will lower in between your legs. Don't hunch your back.

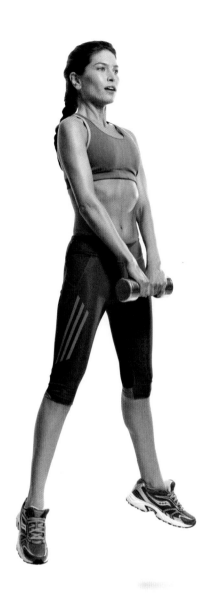

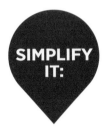

SUPER-CHARGE IT:

There's no need to supercharge this exercise unless you want to work with heavier weight. Make sure your jump is controlled so you land cleanly and don't lose balance.

SIMPLIFY IT:

Try this exercise without weight and concentrate on clean, controlled jumps. You can add weight as you get stronger.

C

Explode upward so you jump off the ground. Keep your arms straight in front of you. When you land, you'll be back in the starting position. Repeat for 60 seconds.

LEG LIFT WITH BAND STRETCH

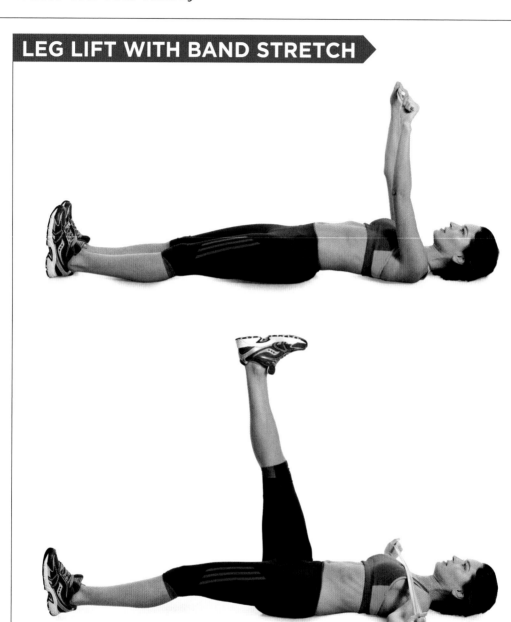

While lying on your back, hold a resistance band up in front of your shoulders. Lift your right leg without bending it until it's straight up. Simultaneously pull your hands until your arms are open wide and the band is stretched across your chest. Hold for a second and then lower your leg and return your arms to the starting position. Alternate leg lifts for 60 seconds.

WEEK

1 2 3 **4**

DAY

1 2 **3** 4 5 6

TODAY'S WORKOUT:

60 SECONDS:
Lateral Glider Lunge with Weight

60 SECONDS:
Torso Twist with Weight

60 SECONDS:
Lateral Glider Lunge with Weight

60 SECONDS:
Torso Twist with Weight

60 SECONDS:
Lateral Glider Lunge with Weight

5 minutes and you're done!

"The more you praise and celebrate your life, the more there is in life to celebrate."

—OPRAH WINFREY

LATERAL GLIDER LUNGE WITH WEIGHT

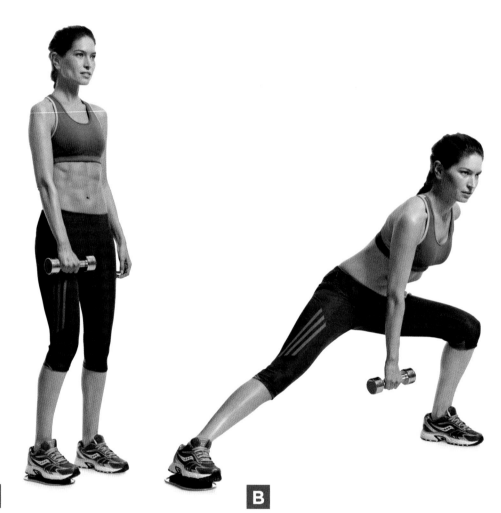

A

Stand with a dumbbell in your right hand. Place a glider or paper plate under your right foot.

B

Keeping your right leg straight and concentrating weight on your right heel, slide the disc out to the side. Bend your left knee as your body lowers and let the weight touch the floor. Hold for a second.

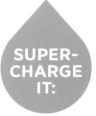

SUPER-CHARGE IT:

After you rise, lift the weight to chest level (an upright row), then press the weight over your head. Hold for a second, then lower and continue as described.

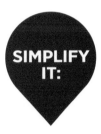

SIMPLIFY IT:

If lowering the weight to the ground is too difficult at first, lower yourself as much as you can without breaking proper form. You can also take out the upright row and simply hold the weight in front of you for the duration of the exercise. As you get stronger, do the exercise as described.

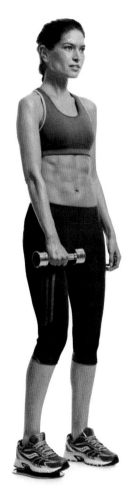

C

Reverse the move, bringing your right foot back toward your center and rising with the weight. Repeat for 30 seconds. Switch sides and continue for 30 seconds.

TORSO TWIST WITH WEIGHT

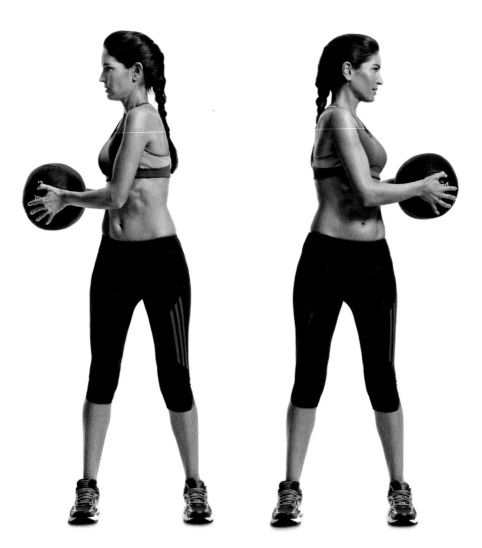

Stand holding a medicine ball (or both ends of a dumbbell) in front of you with your arms bent at 90 degrees. Press your hands toward each other to add arm tension. Twist your torso to the right while keeping your arms at 90 degrees. Without pausing, twist all the way to your left. Continue back and forth for 60 seconds.

60 SECONDS:
Single-Leg
Balance Touch

60 SECONDS:
Single-Arm Plank

60 SECONDS:
Single-Leg
Balance Touch

60 SECONDS:
Single-Arm Plank

60 SECONDS:
Single-Leg
Balance Touch

*5 minutes and
you're done!*

"The most
effective way to
do it, is to do it."
—AMELIA EARHART

SINGLE-LEG BALANCE TOUCH

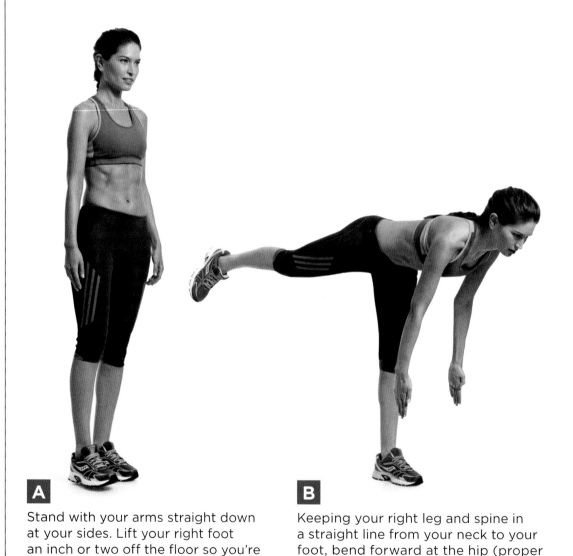

A

Stand with your arms straight down at your sides. Lift your right foot an inch or two off the floor so you're standing on your left foot.

B

Keeping your right leg and spine in a straight line from your neck to your foot, bend forward at the hip (proper form is important). Reach down with your hands and touch your left ankle. Hold for a second.

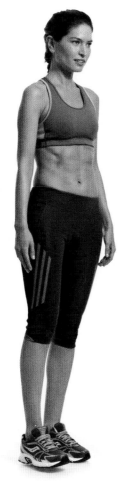

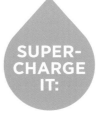

SUPER-CHARGE IT:

After touching your ankle, spread your arms out to the side until they're straight (like a bird's wings). Hold for a second, return your hands back to your left ankle, and continue as described.

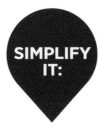

SIMPLIFY IT:

If you have trouble keeping proper form, lower yourself only as far as you can before returning to the starting position. It's important to maintain a straight-through line with your spine and leg.

C

Return to the starting position. Continue for 30 seconds. Switch legs and repeat on the other side for 30 seconds.

SINGLE-ARM PLANK

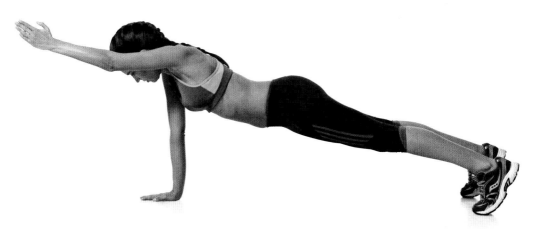

Get into a pushup position. Brace your core and lift your left arm until it's parallel to your left ear. Hold this position for 30 seconds. Switch arms and hold on the other hand for 30 seconds.

TODAY'S WORKOUT:

60 SECONDS:
Burpee with Weight

60 SECONDS:
High Knees with Overhead Hold

60 SECONDS:
Burpee with Weight

60 SECONDS:
High Knees with Overhead Hold

60 SECONDS:
Burpee with Weight

5 minutes and you're done!

"They can because they think they can."

—VIRGIL

BURPEE WITH WEIGHT

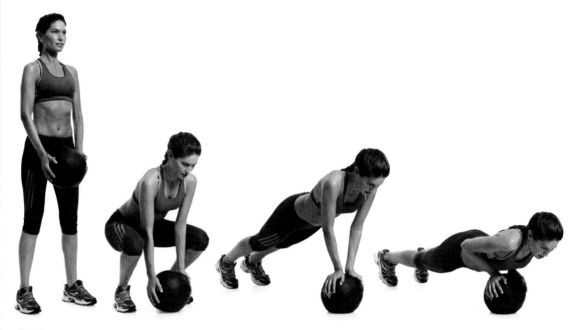

A

Stand with a medicine ball (or two hexagonal dumbbells) in your hands. Squat while lowering the ball in between your legs until it's on the ground.

B

Using the ball (or weights) as your base, jump your feet back so you're in a pushup position. Do a pushup.

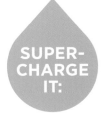

SUPER-CHARGE IT:

When you get into the pushup position, do 2 to 5 pushups. Another idea: After doing a pushup, perform a set of 5 Mountain Climbers (per leg).

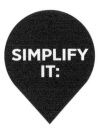

SIMPLIFY IT:

Try the exercise without weight. Add in weight as you get stronger.

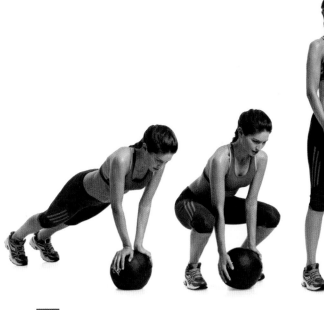

Immediately jump your feet back into a squatting position. Explode upward and jump. Land in the standing position. That's 1 rep. Repeat for 60 seconds.

HIGH KNEES WITH OVERHEAD HOLD

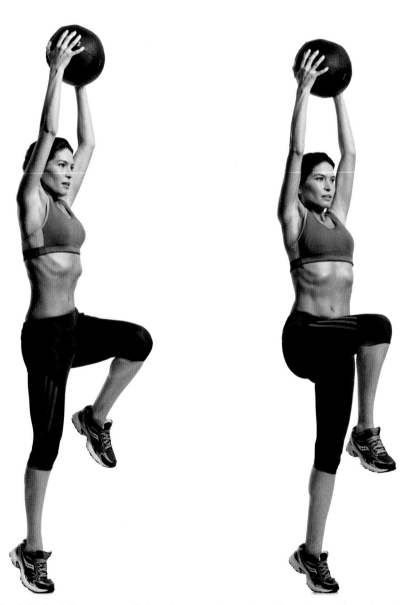

Stand while holding a medicine ball or two dumbbells overhead. While holding the weight up, drive one knee up until it's parallel with your hips. Repeat by alternating legs for 60 seconds. Don't lower the weight until you're finished.

TODAY'S WORKOUT:

60 SECONDS:
Single-Leg Balance with One-Arm Row

60 SECONDS:
Single-Arm Plank with Rotation

60 SECONDS:
Single-Leg Balance with One-Arm Row

60 SECONDS:
Single-Arm Plank with Rotation

60 SECONDS:
Single-Leg Balance with One-Arm Row

5 minutes and you're done!

"Action is the foundational key to all success."

—PABLO PICASSO

SINGLE-LEG BALANCE WITH ONE-ARM ROW

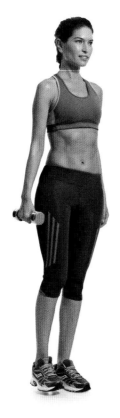

A

Stand with a dumbbell in your right hand, arms at your sides. Lift your right foot an inch or two off the floor so you're standing on your left foot.

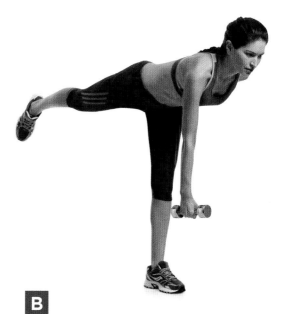

B

Keeping your right leg and spine in a straight line from your neck to your foot, bend forward at the hip (proper form is important). Keep your left (non-dumbbell) arm against your torso. Let your right (dumbbell) arm hang straight to the floor as you bend. Your torso and leg should be parallel with the floor.

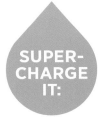

SUPER-CHARGE IT:

In the bottom position, perform a set of 3 rows before returning to the starting position.

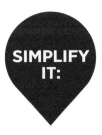

SIMPLIFY IT:

If you have trouble keeping proper form, lower yourself only as far as you can before returning to the starting position. It's important to maintain a straight-through line with your spine and leg.

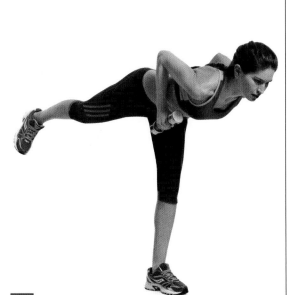

C

While in this position, lift the weight up to your chest. Hold for a second and then lower it back down. Return to the starting position. Repeat for 30 seconds. Switch legs and repeat on the other side for 30 seconds.

SINGLE-ARM PLANK WITH ROTATION

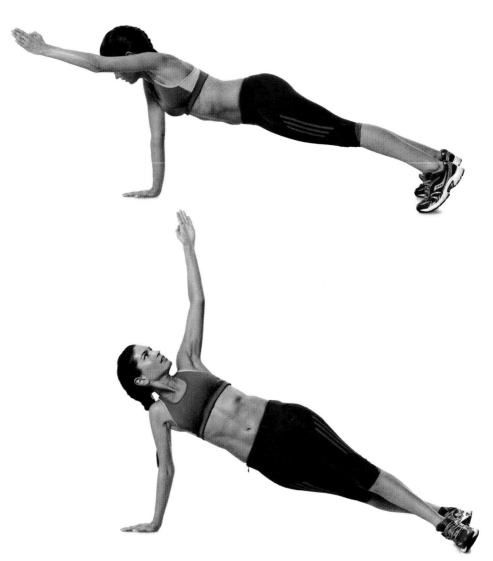

Get into a pushup position. Lift your left arm so it extends straight out in front of you. Using your right arm as a base and keeping your body in a straight line from your neck to your feet, rotate so you go from facing the floor to facing the wall. Reach your extended left hand to the ceiling. Hold for a second. Return to the starting position and alternate sides for 60 seconds.

Congratulations! You did it! Now it's time to monitor your Week 4 progress. This little exercise will keep you focused and accountable. Just answer the following questions:

1. What is your current weight? Use a scale to weigh yourself and also write down your original weight. _____

2. What have you done well this week? What makes you proud?

_____

_____

_____

3. What could you be doing better? _____

_____

_____

4. What's your game plan for Week 5? (see the next chapter for some ideas).

_____

_____

_____

Why I Love Foam Rolling

If you've never heard of foam rolling, don't skip this section. If you have heard of foam rolling, and have even tried it, consider this some positive reinforcement about one of the best things you can do for the health of your muscles and connective tissues. Foam rolling is as basic as it gets: Use a hard Styrofoam roller to massage your tight muscles. Rollers come in various sizes, but a general 36-inch model works just fine.

When you foam-roll, you give yourself a deep-tissue massage. By rolling the hard foam over your thighs, calves, and back, you'll loosen tough connective tissue (like fascia, which stretches over and through many of your muscles and can tighten up) and decrease muscle stiffness. The result? Better flexibility and mobility, and muscles that can function properly. I recommend foam rolling before any workout, but in reality, you can do it anytime. I like to foam-roll while watching TV.

You can find foam rollers at just about any fitness or sports retailer with prices ranging from $12 to $35. (If you don't have one on hand right this second, I've seen people use a basketball or length of PVC pipe in a pinch!) I think it's one of the best investments anyone can make for long-term fitness.

If you've never foam-rolled before, be prepared. It's uncomfortable and can even be painful when you start. *Don't worry! Don't stop!* The more painful it is, the more that muscle needs foam rolling. The good news is that the more you do it, the better it feels. For each muscle that you work, slowly move the roller back and forth over it for 30 seconds. If you hit a really tender spot, pause on it for 5 to 10 seconds.

HAMSTRING ROLL

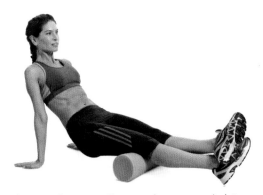

Place a foam roller under your right knee, with your leg straight. Cross your left leg over your right ankle. Put your hands flat on the floor for support. Keep your back naturally arched.

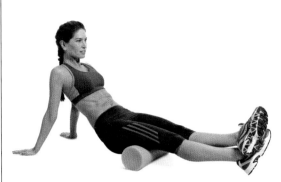

Roll your body forward until the roller reaches your butt. Then roll back and forth. Repeat with the roller under your left thigh. Note: If rolling one leg is too difficult, perform the movement with both legs on the roller.

GLUTE ROLL

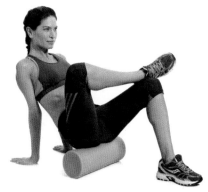

Sit on a foam roller with it positioned on the back of your right thigh, just below your glutes. Cross your right leg over the front of your left thigh. Put your hands flat on the floor for support.

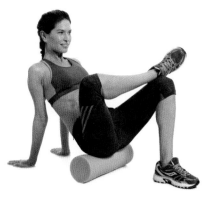

Roll your body forward until the roller reaches your lower back. Then roll back and forth. Repeat with the roller under your left glute.

ILIOTIBIAL-BAND ROLL

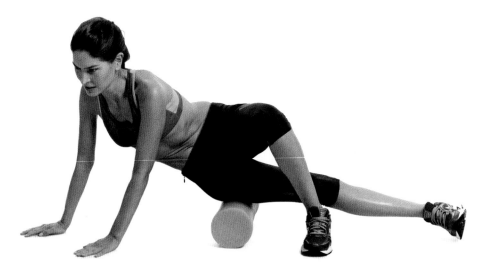

Lie on your right side and place your right hip on a foam roller. Put your hands on the floor for support. Cross your left leg over your right and place your left foot flat on the floor.

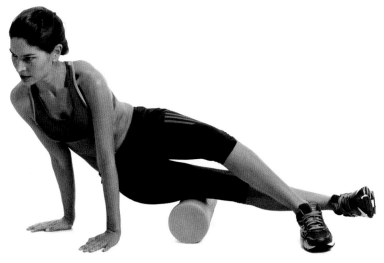

Roll your body forward until the roller reaches your knee. Then roll back and forth. Lie on your left side and repeat with the roller under your left hip. (If this becomes too easy over time, place one leg on top of the other instead of bracing one on the floor.)

CALF ROLL

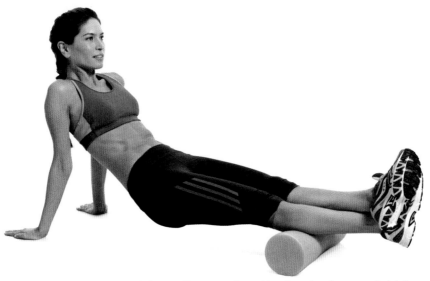

Place a foam roller under your right ankle, with your right leg straight. Cross your left leg over your right ankle. Put your hands flat on the floor for support and keep your back naturally arched.

Roll your body forward until the roller reaches the back of your right knee. Then roll back and forth. Repeat with the roller under your left calf. (If this is too hard, perform the movement with both legs on the roller.)

QUADRICEP-AND-HIP-FLEXOR ROLL

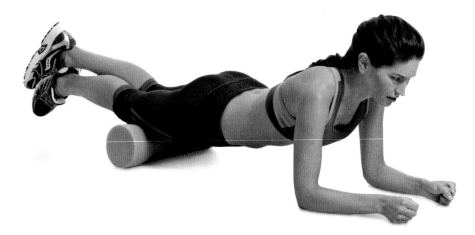

Lie facedown on the floor with a foam roller positioned above your right knee. Cross your left leg over your right ankle and place your elbows on the floor for support.

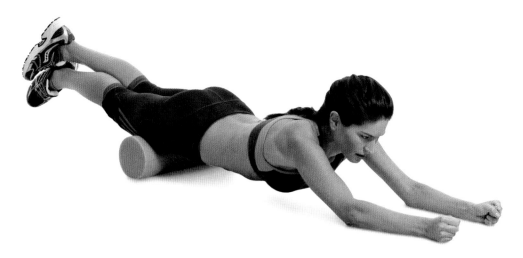

Roll your body backward until the roller reaches the top of your right thigh. Then roll back and forth. Repeat with the roller under your left thigh. (If that's too hard, perform the movement with both thighs on the roller.)

LOWER-BACK ROLL

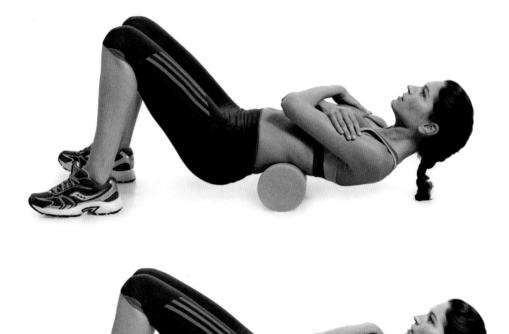

Lie faceup with a foam roller under your midback. Cross your arms over your chest. Your knees should be bent, with your feet flat on the floor. Raise your hips off the floor slightly. Roll back and forth over your lower back.

UPPER-BACK ROLL

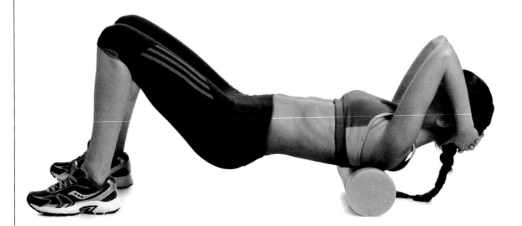

Lie faceup with a foam roller under your midback, at the bottom of your shoulder blades. Clasp your hands behind your head and pull your elbows toward each other. Raise your hips off the floor slightly.

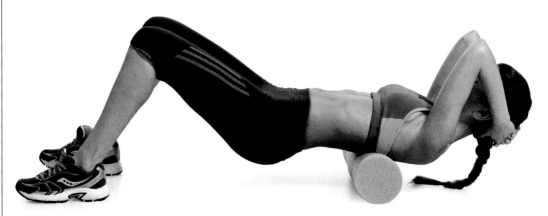

Slowly lower your back downward, so that your upper back bends over the foam roller. Raise back to the start and roll forward a couple of inches—so that the roller sits higher under your upper back—and repeat. Roll forward one more time and do it again. That's 1 rep.

SHOULDER-BLADE ROLL

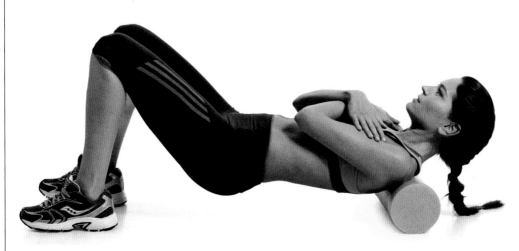

Lie faceup with a foam roller under your upper back, at the tops of your shoulder blades. Cross your arms over your chest. Your knees should be bent with your feet flat on the floor.

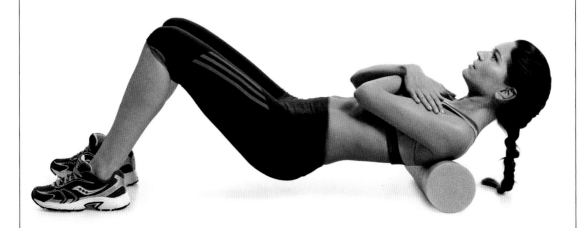

Raise your hips so they're slightly elevated off the floor. Roll back and forth over your shoulder blades and your mid- and upper back.

Chapter
5

Inches Off!
Your
Tummy
Eating
Guidelines

"Tell me what you eat, and I will tell you who you are."

—BRILLAT-SAVARIN

EAT TO LOSE WEIGHT—
THE SCIENTIFIC SECRET

Over the years, I've heard a lot of metaphors for people and eating.

"You're an engine—but you must put the right fuel in the gas tank!"

"Building muscle is like building a house—you need the right raw materials and a solid foundation!"

"Your body is a temple—and you've been treating it like a garbage dump!"

They're all pretty accurate. And they all colorfully illustrate the real truth at work between the food on our fork and the urge to fill our bellies with it: If you eat healthy foods in sensible portions, your body will respond by working and looking better. Unfortunately, the reality is that the way most of us have been taught to eat—even when dieting—sets us up to get fatter. The average person consumes too much sugar and too many refined carbohydrates.

That's what this chapter is all about—consuming the right fuel (the right foods) so our engines run optimally.

It's actually pretty simple if you can understand two concepts. First, you must eat foods that don't spike insulin. I'll explain this in detail later in this chapter—but just know that insulin is the hormone that drives fat storage and tells your body to hang on to fat you already have. Keeping it low keeps fat melting off your body. Simple. Second, not all calories count. Again, I'll get into this in detail in the paragraphs below—just remember that only Sugar Calories (the calories from carbs and sugar) count, because these are the calories that spike insulin. See the link? Count and limit the insulin-spiking calories and you'll lose weight.

This chapter on food is just as important as the exercise section of the book, and it essentially follows the same line of thinking that I introduced with exercise. Conventional wisdom about dieting and weight loss is misguided; to lose weight

YOUR INCHES OFF! **EDGE**
The Inches Off! eating plan is simple and straightforward.

- This is a no-deprivation diet.

- You'll learn how to eat all your favorite foods.

- You'll count only the calories that count.

- You'll solve the issues behind emotional eating.

- You'll fill your body with the right foods needed to build muscle and burn fat.

we need to get back to our roots and eat like our ancestors did. That's how I've designed the Inches Off! eating guidelines. On the following pages you'll find all the tools needed to succeed. In the end, it is so simple:

- The right foods can prevent your body from storing fat.

- The right foods can also help your body burn fat.

- Not all calories count.

Later in this chapter you will find a sample meal planner, and I provide food lists in Chapter 6 (with all the Sugar Calories already calculated for you!). This is so you can create healthy meals that work as a companion to your Inches Off! workouts—helping you see results even faster. For more options, menus, and recipes, please visit my Web site at jorgecruise.com.

In our society, we are told to eat a diet that is around 50 percent carbohydrates—and if we want to lose weight, we're told to simply cut calories. We're told this by just about every public health agency out there, including the USDA, the American Dietetic Association, and the National Institutes of Health, to name

just a few. Most of our diets reflect this recommended amount of carbs, and many of us are consuming too many calories from sugars and high fructose corn syrup. So what happens? You guessed it: Surplus energy is stored as fat, and that's why a majority of the population is overweight or obese. The problem is, we're eating way too many insulin-spiking foods and getting way too many calories from carbs and sugars.

This is a new development for humans, and just as most exercise isn't designed to work with the way our bodies are biologically adapted to function, most recommendations for eating do not work with the way we were designed to eat. Think about it: Before we learned how to farm and make things like refined sugar or white flour, humans simply didn't eat any sugar unless they got it naturally from tubers (low-sugar potato-like vegetables), fruit (along with the vitamins and fiber fruit also provides, unlike candy bars) or perhaps honey (if they braved the bees). Back then, humans weren't fat, and they didn't have most of the obesity-related diseases that we do today. Their diets were primarily protein, fat, and green leafy vegetables. If something was going to kill us before our time,

WHAT IS A **SUGAR CALORIE?**

Any carbohydrate food (including all sugars) is a Sugar Calorie. This is because all carbohydrates and sugars are broken down into glucose (the body's sugar) at a molecular level.

it generally had teeth. So history has shown that we really don't need all that much sugar to live an active, productive life. Today our diets are saturated in these fat-adding Sugar Calories.

If you eat a diet low in Sugar Calories, as our ancestors did, you avoid insulin spikes. If you avoid insulin spikes, you won't be storing fat. And even better—if you eat intelligently, consuming healthy foods in sensible amounts, you'll lose fat.

THE SCIENTIFIC SECRET TO WEIGHT LOSS—
INSULIN DRIVES FAT, AND NOT ALL CALORIES COUNT

What I'm about to share with you took me 10 years to figure out. If you want to lose weight, there are two critical keys that will unlock the secret: Lower insulin and eat the right amounts of the right calories.

So How Does Insulin Make You Fat?

Insulin is the hormone that helps push fat into fat cells, so decades of research—and common sense—show that if no insulin is present, fat cannot be stored. We've heard mixed messages over the years about weight loss: calories in, calories out, exercise more, eat less. These theories are misleading because our bodies are a lot more complicated than simple math. If you understand how insulin works with your body, you'll understand a new way of

eating that will make weight loss easier than ever.

So how does insulin make us fat? Insulin is the master hormone in your body that tells it what to do with the fuel (food) that you consume. If what you're eating or drinking is high in Sugar Calories, the sugar in your blood will spike, which triggers insulin production. Insulin then tells your body to store away the food as fat and to hang on to the fat your body already has. On the other hand, if what you eat is protein or fat, it doesn't raise your blood sugar and insulin isn't triggered, so your body isn't told to store the fuel as fat or to hold on to the fat that is already stored—it actually does the opposite. Now, I'm simplifying this so it's easy to comprehend, but the bottom line is that Sugar Calories drive insulin, and insulin drives fat accumulation and storage.

Track Only the Calories That Count

What exactly is a calorie? We see these numbers tied to all the foods and drinks we consume; we hear recommendations of how many we should have (the USDA bases all of our recommended daily nutrients on a 2,000-calorie diet); we're told that if we want to lose weight, we should cut these calories and burn more off through exercise. But what are these pesky little numbers? Since 2011, as part of President Barack Obama's health care initiative, all large restaurant chains in the nation are required to include calorie counts on menus and drive-thru signs. This same legislation also requires that vending machines post calories. The problem with these labels is that they include the total calories a food contains for all its nutrients, but not all these calories count when it comes to weight loss. And that's where we get sidetracked; we try to count all calories, instead of focusing on the calories that will cause weight gain.

So back to the question at hand, what is a calorie? According to the people who study such things, a calorie is a unit of measurement for heat; in science, a calorie is defined as the unit of heat required to raise 1 gram of water 1 degree Celsius. How does that relate to food? Back in the late 1800s, when scientists needed to figure out the calorie counts in foods, they would literally light them on fire, then put them in water, and then check the change in water temperature to determine the calories in a certain food. So if the burnt food raised the temperature of the water by 5 degrees, it would equal 5 calories, and so on. What is actually being measured is how much energy is lost to the fire. The theory was that this was the same energy that would be "lost" to your body if you ate the food.

Today scientists and chemists use a more precise measuring process to determine calories that takes into account the specific amounts of moisture, fat, carbohydrates, and protein in foods, but the description above paints the general picture. From all this measuring, scientists today have determined that:

- 1 gram of fat contains 9 calories.

- 1 gram of protein contains 4 calories.

- 1 gram of carbohydrates contains 4 calories (sugar is counted in carbohydrate grams).

Therefore, the number of calories in any food item is equal to its grams of fat × 9 + grams of protein × 4 + grams of carbohydrates × 4. For example, in a chocolate kiss, which contains 1.3 grams of fat, 0 gram of protein, and 3.6 grams of carbohydrates, the equation would go as follows:

$$\frac{\begin{array}{l}(1.3 \text{ g fat})(9 \text{ cal/g}) \\ + (0 \text{ g protein})(4 \text{ cal/g}) \\ + (3.6 \text{ g carbohydrates})(4 \text{ cal/g})\end{array}}{26.1 \text{ calories. \textbf{TA-DA!}}}$$

The recommendations to cut calories come from the folks who believe that burning off calories works much the same way as setting food on fire. This would be nice and simple, but the fact is that our bodies don't work like an incinerator that just burns up whatever fuel we put in it. Our bodies have a much more complex relationship with the food we eat. To illustrate what I mean, let's compare one normal-size Reese's Peanut Butter Cup (105 calories) to a handful of dry-roasted peanuts that equal the same calorie count (about 18 peanuts). If you believe that a calorie is a calorie is a calorie, then these two foods should be identical, but it's not that simple. The candy is composed of 12 grams of carbs, which equals 48 calories of carbohydrates or Sugar Calories (remember a carbohydrate gram is worth 4 calories). These Sugar Calories are the calories that spike insulin and cause fat accumulation and resistance to releasing fat from the body. The peanuts, on the other hand, have just 3.9 grams of carbs, which equals 15.6 calories—not enough to cause a spike in insulin, which means that you won't store fat from that food. The peanut butter cup has more than three times the weight-causing calories in the peanuts.

If you eat a diet that is composed mostly of Sugar Calories, you will set yourself up to gain weight or you will maintain the excess weight that you want to lose—even if you cut overall calories. In contrast, the calories in proteins and fats won't spike blood sugar or insulin, which is why these calories don't count in the same way—in fact, they help your body burn fat as fuel and let go of stored fat. I call these foods Freebies.

The Inches Off! 5-Minute Fitness Formula works in tandem with this style of eating to give you even better results. How? The food acts as muscle-building fuel, and the workouts help you build

A HELPFUL HINT: INVEST YOUR SUGAR CALORIES WISELY

If you rack up any Sugar Calories during the day—on this plan you're allowed 100 each day—my advice is to make those calories as nutritionally dense as possible. This means that even though your blood sugar may rise when you eat these foods, at least you'll be getting a nice boost of vitamins, minerals, and other good things. Here are some examples:

- Blueberries and strawberries are a better Sugar Calorie investment than a slice of whole wheat bread.

- Black beans (or any legume) are a better Sugar Calorie investment than potatoes.

- Adding fresh fruit and a dash of honey to plain Greek yogurt is a better Sugar Calorie investment than the same calorie load in ice cream.

You see my point? Sugar Calories don't have to be a total supervillain if you choose intelligently.

that new muscle. Well, guess what? Muscle is metabolically active tissue, and one of its functions is to help process blood glucose. The more muscle you have, the easier it is for your body to process sugar. A combination of good eating and dedicated exercising will prevent your body from storing fat and help it burn off the fat you have.

"SO . . . HOW MANY SUGAR CALORIES
CAN I EAT?"

That's a great question. On the Inches Off! program, you can eat up to 100 Sugar Calories a day. This virtually guarantees that you won't spike insulin and your body will maintain a healthy, steady-state blood sugar all day long. If 100 doesn't sound like a lot, well, "a lot" is relative. As you'll see, you'll still be eating "a lot," since there are plenty of yummy, zero–Sugar Calorie foods to choose from. In fact, when it comes to these foods, I have just one piece of advice . . .

Chase the Freebies!

Now that you understand the basics of how the wrong foods can sabotage your eating plan, you're probably starting to wonder what the "right" foods are. Well, I want you to think "Freebies!" On the Inches Off! plan, Freebies are foods that have no Sugar Calories, meaning they cause little or no insulin spiking. You'll see lots of Freebies in the sample planner on page 161 and the calculated food lists in the next chapter. The more Freebies you work into your daily meals, the less insulin you'll produce and the less fat you'll store. Not to mention, you'll never be hungry!

Meats, fish, fats, and some dairy are a few examples of Freebies. Protein is a big deal on the Inches Off! plan, since it is essential for building muscle, and we want your body primed to do that with every workout. But there's another set of Freebies that are even more important; so important, in fact, that they are still considered Freebies even though they contain mostly carbohydrates. What is this mystery group?

Vegetables!

I hope you make Freebie vegetables part of every meal. They're loaded with nutrients you need, as well as fiber, and they work wonderfully with other Freebies like meat and fish. For example, if you have a lunch of grilled chicken on a bed of greens with a dash of olive oil vinaigrette, that's a plate of Freebies that

WHAT IS A **FREEBIE FOOD?**

Any food that keeps insulin levels low, including proteins, fats, some dairy, Freebie Vegetables, and Freebie Flours (see pages 170–171).

will keep you feeling full—and nourished—all afternoon. (Eggs are a Freebie, so imagine the breakfast possibilities pairing eggs with various vegetable combos.)

Now, it's true that some vegetables contain natural sugar and can affect your insulin response (though not nearly as much as, say, a candy bar). But broccoli and many other vegetables are so nutritious and good for you, I'm calling them Freebies.

I'm also making the call right here: Tomatoes are Freebies. They're so nutritious (I really like the lycopene for prostate health) and versatile (they're great in salads and protein dishes) that I line them up with vegetables—even though they are technically a fruit.

Fruits, on the other hand, are not Freebies. But I'll be honest: Using your daily Sugar Calorie allotment for fruit is one of the best eating choices you can make. Berries, for example, are a delicious snack—and one of the healthiest foods out there. So be smart about your Sugar Calories (see "A Helpful Hint: Invest Your Sugar Calories Wisely" on page 157), and you'll eat like a champion.

How It Works

As I explained above, what the new science about weight loss has taught me, and I'm now teaching you, is that you don't have to count calories from protein and fat, just those derived from carbohydrates—and that's how I've designed the Inches Off! eating guidelines. What does that mean? Let's look at the nutrient label for

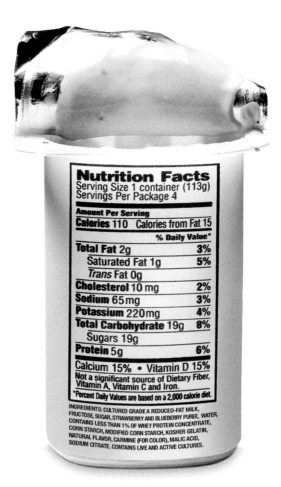

Nutrition Facts
Serving Size 1 container (113g)
Servings Per Package 4

Amount Per Serving	
Calories 110	Calories from Fat 15

	% Daily Value*
Total Fat 2g	3%
Saturated Fat 1g	5%
Trans Fat 0g	
Cholesterol 10 mg	2%
Sodium 65 mg	3%
Potassium 220 mg	4%
Total Carbohydrate 19g	8%
Sugars 19g	
Protein 5g	6%

Calcium 15% • Vitamin D 15%

Not a significant source of Dietary Fiber, Vitamin A, Vitamin C and Iron.

*Percent Daily Values are based on a 2,000 calorie diet.

INGREDIENTS: CULTURED GRADE A REDUCED-FAT MILK, FRUCTOSE, SUGAR, STRAWBERRY AND BLUEBERRY PUREE, WATER, CONTAINS LESS THAN 1% OF WHEY PROTEIN CONCENTRATE, CORN STARCH, MODIFIED CORN STARCH, KOSHER GELATIN, NATURAL FLAVOR, CARMINE (FOR COLOR), MALIC ACID, SODIUM CITRATE. CONTAINS LIVE AND ACTIVE CULTURES.

yogurt here. It tells you that one container equals 110 calories—but not so fast. When we look at the breakdown of calories, realizing that protein and fat calories don't count, the yogurt really has 76 Sugar Calories, not 110. How do I get that number? See the formula below.

19 grams of carbs in yogurt
x 4 calories per carb gram
_____
76 Sugar Calories

Sugar Calories are calculated by multiplying the number of total carbohydrates by 4 calories per gram.

Since we know that the calories in the yogurt from protein and fat don't count because they actually help you lose weight, we don't count them. By focusing your diet on foods that help you stay under my recommended 100 Sugar Calories, you can lose weight while still satisfying your body with the Freebie foods—proteins and fats and a few other goodies. Proteins and fats are the most satisfying, slowly digesting, non-insulin-stimulating foods—so filling your food plan with them, along with vegetables, is the best way to lose weight. In the next chapter you'll see extensive food lists that will clue you in on the foods you can enjoy and the ones you need to avoid by highlighting the Sugar Calories. Keep in mind that the Freebies will supercharge your weight loss because they keep insulin at low levels, which means you can burn fat at higher rates for more hours of each day. These are the foods that should be the foundation of your daily eating plan.

Ready to eat? In the Appendix on page 203, I've provided complete, "Done-For-You" meal planners that will accelerate your weight loss by telling you exactly what you need to eat each day. It couldn't be simpler. Do you want to create your own meals? Go to JorgeCruise.com for a free blank meal planner. Basically you'll be marking down your Sugar Calories and keeping them under 100 per day. All you have to do is use my calculated food lists in the next chapter or look up the carb grams in a food and multiply them by 4. Choose the healthiest Sugar Calories and save those with the highest levels of sugars and refined flours for special treat days. In addition, make sure you include plenty of Freebies—that's the fastest way to lose weight.

Don't forget to be smart about snacks. Snacks are best used as a way to stay satisfied from one meal to the next. Nuts and cheese are the perfect choices here because they are almost exclusively protein or fat based, with little to no sugar or carbs.

"SO . . . WHAT CAN I HAVE AS A DESSERT?"

Once a day, whenever you prefer, you can have one treat. (I like mine after dinner.) You'll see the dessert box on the meal planner. The key here is to not allow a treat to turn into a feast. I'm talking about having a small portion of something you love. My favorite treats are dark chocolate and a glass of red wine. For a lot of us, it's worth it to save a few Sugar Calories for last.

THE INCHES OFF! SAMPLE MEAL PLANNER:
WHAT DOES A DAY OF EATING LOOK LIKE?

MEAL: Breakfast	SUGAR CALORIES (carb grams x 4)
2 scrambled eggs	Freebie
3 slices turkey bacon, extra lean	Freebie
MEAL: Snack	
1 string cheese	Freebie
MEAL: Lunch	
1 slice Food For Life Ezekiel 4:9 Sprouted Grain Bread	60
1 slice (1 oz) Swiss cheese	Freebie
3 oz cooked 85% lean ground turkey patty	Freebie
3 lettuce leaves	Freebie
2 slices tomato	Freebie
1 Tbsp mayonnaise	Freebie
MEAL: Snack	
11 dry-roasted almonds	Freebie
MEAL: Dinner	
3–4 oz grilled chicken or fish	Freebie
1 cup mixed greens	Freebie
1 cup chopped tomato and spinach	Freebie
2 Tbsp olive oil and vinegar	Freebie
MEAL: Dessert	
1 glass (5 oz) cabernet sauvignon wine	14
DAILY TOTAL	**74 Sugar Calories**

WHAT ABOUT **WATER?**

I recommend drinking at least eight glasses (8 ounces each) a day, but again, get in touch with your body. When you feel thirsty, drink. Staying hydrated keeps your body systems running well, can reduce or relieve headaches, and enhances energy. And a glass of water can do away with false hunger.

WHEN SHOULD I **EAT?**

A lot has been said in the last decade about eating five or six small meals during the day. The thinking was that more frequent, smaller meals would help keep your metabolism stoked throughout the day and also keep you from feeling hungry. Some research supports this, while other studies show that eating less frequently throughout the day might be better. I say that you should listen to your own individual body wisdom.

We all experience important hunger signals, but because of years of following diets and "shoulds" about eating, most of us eat according to some rule, not because our bodies inform us we are hungry. I want you to get back in touch with the healthy signals your body gives off that tell you when you are truly body hungry, satisfied, or full (different from satisfied). It's important to get back in touch with this because it will help you eat what your body needs, when it needs it—and

stop you from eating more than your body really wants.

Throughout the day, check in with your body. When you start thinking about food, ask yourself, "Am I really hungry, or am I just mind hungry?" True body hunger has a sharp signal that often comes with stomach growling, hunger pangs, and slight dizziness, while mind hunger is a desire for food devoid of any physical sensations of hunger (often triggered by stress, boredom, or depression). Body hunger is also often accompanied by a desire for a specific food. So the second question to ask yourself, after you've determined that you are really feeling hungry, is "what food do I want?" Hot or cold, spicy or sweet, soft or crunchy, and so on. If you have a meal that you truly desire, you will be much more satisfied than if you choose to eat what you think you should. As you are eating your meal pay attention to what you are eating so you are able to detect the soft signal that feeling satisfied gives off. This happens before you notice that

THE MOTIVATOR STOP BEING TO BUSY TO EAT.

Skipped lunch? Of course you're going to chow down on unhealthy amounts later. Most people make poor eating decisions when they are missing meals—their blood sugar drops and then the cravings creep in. Keep your cravings at bay with a healthy snack between regular full meals. (See page 169 for an entire chapter of great ideas!) I always try to eat something every 3 hours or so.

you've had one bite too many, but you must pay attention to catch it. Don't beat yourself up if you miss it and eat until you feel a bit too full. Use this as a lesson. Take notice of what "too full" feels like; it will help you get in touch with the subtle signal satiation gives.

That's what makes the Inches Off! meal planner so easy to use: You can eat whenever your body is hungry. There are no set times that you must have meals. Just follow the directions outlined in this chapter. If you want to portion out those meals into smaller, more frequent meals, feel free. Or you can have three traditional meals with snacks. It's up to you. Just remember, 100 Sugar Calories is your limit for the day.

RULES FOR
SMART EATING

Besides putting the right foods on your plate, you should follow a couple of additional rules for optimal weight-loss success.

Try to eat meals and snacks at **the same time every day.** People who are trying to break bad eating habits tend to stress about how much they eat and when they should eat. I want you to break the spell food has cast over you. Food is fuel, and fueling is routine. Think of mealtime and snack time as simple mileposts in your day, not grand showdowns between you and your willpower. It's just food. If you establish a routine and eat at roughly the same time each day, eating stops being a big, stressful deal, and it becomes just another step toward your goals.

Stop eating 3 hours before bed. Finally, shut the refrigerator and put an imaginary CLOSED sign in your kitchen 3 hours before you go to bed (or maybe even a literal sign). When you eat 2 to 3 hours before going to sleep, you take too much food to bed with you, and your digestive system keeps you awake as it breaks down your food. Though you may actually be able to fall asleep, you won't sleep deeply as your body digests. And you need deep sleep for your body to

THE MOTIVATOR ALWAYS FOCUS ON THE SMALLER NUMBER.

Big numbers are scary. So go low. For example: When you're starting out on a weight-loss plan, never say, "I want to lose X number of pounds." That's a big number and can seem out of reach. Start out saying, "I want to have a great week and lose a couple of pounds." Then, as your progress builds and you cross over the halfway mark to your goal, switch it around: "Only X pounds to go!" Smaller numbers always seem more achievable.

truly rest and recover from exercise. I want your body rebuilding itself as you sleep, not breaking down food. I promise you will feel more energized and alive when you wake!

THE SAFETY BELT
SYSTEM

With the help of millions of online and personal clients, I've come up with the following five safety belts to help you prevent random acts of overeating.

Safety Belt #1: The Audio Loop

This safety belt works a lot like self-hypnosis. For this one, you will create a digital or audiotape that you will listen to frequently to help protect yourself from overeating. To make your audio loop, come up with very short answers to the following questions.

1. What will I lose in my life if I don't take care of myself? For example, you might write, "If I fail to take good care of myself, I could lose my health, my energy, and my relationships."

2. What will I gain when I get healthy? Here you might write, "If I stick with the program, I'll be able to show off my belly, feel more confident, and live longer."

Keep your answers short. Reading them out loud should take less than 30 seconds. You will then record your answers on a tape or digital recorder (a lot of smartphones have a voice memo feature). When you are recording, play dramatic music softly in the background. I suggest using scary background music, such as the theme to *Jaws*, for the first

THE MOTIVATOR CHANGE ONE WORD.

When most people start a weight-loss plan, they'll tell their friends, "I want to lose X pounds," or "I want to look better/get back in shape/feel good naked." Here's one small tweak: Go from "I want" to "I will." Think about it. When you want something, there's always that little voice in the back of your head that says you can't have it. Our society is programmed for instant gratification. You say, "I want new clothes," and you can get them right away if you have a credit card (though I don't recommend racking up debt). But if you say, "I want to lose weight," well, you can't put that on a credit card. It takes time and effort. You might have doubts.

Well, erase them. From now on, forget "I want." Say, "I will lose X pounds; I will look better; I will get back in shape; I will feel good naked!" You won't have a doubt in your mind. And neither will anyone else.

question and inspiring background music, such as the theme to *Chariots of Fire*, for the second question. Make two recordings—one for home and the other for travel (stored on an iPod, for example).

Listen to your audio loop over and over again. It works a lot like a favorite song. Think of a song you've heard played over and over on the radio. After a while, you can hear it in your head without the song being on. That's the power of repetition, and that's what this is all about.

The repetition will ingrain these concepts in your mind, helping to bolster your motivation to stick with the plan. For many years, scientists have known that repeated positive affirmations can help to dramatically improve health. As far back as the early 1900s, a scientist named Émile Coué told his patients to say to themselves, "Every day in every way, I am getting better and better," 20 times each day. If regular positive thoughts can improve your health, just imagine what they can do for your motivation to tone your belly!

Safety Belt #2: Power Quotes

I love inspiring quotations. (You'll find a few in this book!) To me, there's nothing like reading the perfect quote at just the right moment to inspire me to eat right and stick to my fitness routines. That's why I suggest you create a bunch of business cards with power quotes on them. That way, no matter where you find yourself, you can always whip out a card and read a quote to help inspire you to

success. To get started, search through quotation books or Web sites and jot down some quotes that you feel will really help fuel your motivation. These don't have to be quotes from famous people. You can jot down sayings from bumper stickers, T-shirts, greeting cards, or even the casual motivational comments of friends or family. Type your quotes into a word-processing program and print them out onto business cards. (You can purchase perforated cards at an office supply store such as Staples, along with computer software that will help you easily print the quotes onto them.)

Once you've made your cards, laminate them and carry them with you. Look at your cards whenever you need a boost. For example, one of my clients carries a card with a quote from her husband. When she was struggling with an issue at work, he remarked, "Temptation resisted is a true measure of character." The comment struck her so much that she put it on a business card and carries it around with her, using it for a positive boost in any challenging situation.

Another helpful tip: Every night before bed, e-mail a power quote from your personal e-mail to your work e-mail. You'll see it first thing in the morning at work, when you need it most!

Safety Belt #3: Before-and-After Poster

One of my clients placed a photo of herself at her highest weight ever on her fridge. Next to it, she put a photo of herself at her lowest weight ever. Whenever she feels tempted to raid the fridge—a classic weak spot—she sees the photos and thinks, "Who do I want to be, the fat person on the left or the sexy and fit one on the right?" Unless she is physically hungry, she always chooses the sexy and fit one and walks away from the fridge.

If you don't have an "after" photo of yourself, you can use a photo of a healthy model whom you'd like to emulate. Or you can cover your fridge with photos of beautiful bellies cut from magazines. Use whatever images will help you remember your goal.

Safety Belt #4: Grab-and-Go Food List

You're most likely to eat unhealthy foods when you feel stressed or hurried. But you can avoid this problem with a little preparation. Take a moment to brainstorm a number of quick and healthy breakfasts, lunches, dinners, snacks, and treats. For example, you might keep a few frozen dinners on hand or grab a no- or low-sugar meal-replacement shake for a meal. Keep them where you need them—at home, at work, or in a small cooler you bring along in the car for long trips.

Write down as many grab-and-go meals as possible and then post your list on the fridge. This also will help make grocery shopping easier because you can consult your grab-and-go list to see what you need from the store.

Safety Belt #5: The Home Run

This is so simple, yet so powerful. I recommend that you set jorgecruise.com or facebook.com/jorgecruisefan as your home page on your computer at work and at home. Whenever you go onto the Internet, my site will come up and you'll get a great reminder of your weight-loss commitment and all of the positive progress you've already made. As one of my clients says, "When I am at work, I just turn my computer on and see Jorge's face and I feel like he is watching me, and I wouldn't sabotage myself if he were physically here with me!"

THE POWER OF **THREE**

I've provided you with a variety of safety belts. I want you to pick three that you

THE MOTIVATOR DON'T "DIET."

Swap out the word *diet*—which is a loaded word associated with failure in so many ways—with something positive like, "I'm challenging myself to be in the best shape ever." It gets rid of the negativity and skepticism surrounding that four-letter word.

feel will help keep you on track. If you want to use more, that's great. But three is the minimum.

Your three safety belts will help you stick to your plan, eating nutritionally rather than emotionally. Bottom line: If you eat nutritionally, you will create lean muscle. If you eat emotionally, you will create fat. The choice is yours.

Right now, my challenge to you is to choose to eat nutritionally. And to help you overcome emotional eating, use your top three safety belts, but also make sure to come and visit me at jorgecruise.com or facebook.com /jorgecruisefan. There you will meet additional people to support you and help accelerate your weight loss. Before you know it, you will look and feel more beautiful and sexy than you ever have before.

CHOOSE YOUR **SAFETY BELTS**

I want you to firmly commit to using the Safety Belt System by writing down your three safety belts—and how you will use each one—in the space provided.

The three safety belts I will use are:

1. _____

2. _____

3. _____

Here is how I will incorporate each one into my life:

1. _____

2. _____

3. _____

167

"One cannot think well, love well, sleep well, if one has not dined well."

—VIRGINIA WOOLF

To keep your life simple, I've calculated the Sugar Calories for many common foods and put them into easy-to-read lists below. Remember, you calculate Sugar Calories by multiplying the number of carbohydrate grams by 4. Since virtually all nutrition labels are available online at various Web sites, such as calorieking.com, you can always figure out the carbohydrate grams and calculate your own Sugar Calories practically anywhere.

The way it works is easy: You have 100 Sugar Calories a day to choose from, and you can partition them any way you like. As I've said before, I recommend that you add as many Freebies—foods that have zero Sugar Calories—into your daily diet as you can. These are the foods that will fill you up and keep you fueled without causing a blood sugar/insulin spike and, as a result, a fat storage spree around your middle.

This is not a complete list by any means; feel free to look up the nutrition information of many more foods online.

Please note that the calories in the lists below account for just the Sugar Calories, which I've calculated for you—so you don't have to do the work.

FREEBIES

I'm listing Freebies first. The more you incorporate these foods into your day, the easier it will be for you to keep your daily Sugar Calories under 100. Happy eating!

PROTEINS—0 SUGAR CALORIES

Animal proteins are extremely low in carbohydrates, but it's important to exercise care when choosing lunch meats, sausages, hot dogs, or other types of processed meats. Even bacon can have lots of additives and sugar—so read ingredient labels and try to select processed meats that have no added sugars and less than 2 grams of carbohydrates per serving. If they're available to you, the best choices are organic meats, which are free of pesticides and hormones.

Poultry

Chicken breast, leg, thigh, wing

Cornish hen

Lean ground turkey

Turkey breast

Turkey bacon

Turkey burger

Eggs

Chicken (brown or white)

Duck

Egg whites

Goose

Seafood

Catfish	Halibut	Sardines
Clams	Lobster	Scallops
Cod	Mahi-mahi	Shrimp
Crab	Orange roughy	Sole
Flounder	Oysters	Swordfish
	Salmon	Tilapia

WHAT ARE **FREEBIE FLOURS?**

Foods made with white, whole wheat, and other grain-based flours contain high levels of carbohydrates that will quickly eat up your Sugar Calories, spike your levels of insulin, and lead to weight gain and belly fat. Fortunately, I've discovered three fantastic Freebie Flours that have zero Sugar Calories and can be used to make muffins, cakes, pancakes, chips, crackers, and breads. They can also work as breading for fried foods. Today, these flours are available at health food stores and many grocery stores. Not only will these Freebie Flours accelerate your weight loss, they are full of nutrients, antioxidants, and fiber and are gluten free.

COCONUT FLOUR. Full of fiber and low in carbohydrates, this flour makes a great replacement breading for fried chicken and other fried foods. Coconut has also been shown to raise levels of healthy cholesterol. It creates a wonderful crust and has a natural nutty sweetness to it. Coconut flour also makes great muffins, cakes, and breads. Because it is high in fiber, it is extremely absorbent, so you only need ¼ cup for every 1 cup of flour.

FLAX FLOUR. This powerhouse of nutrients, also called flaxseed meal, contains high levels of natural antioxidants, fiber, and healthy omega-3 fatty acids that have been shown to improve hair growth, promote younger-looking skin, reduce risk of cancers and diabetes, protect against heart disease, relieve menopausal symptoms, promote healthy bowel movements, and improve your immune system. Flaxseed flour makes a great nutty-tasting replacement for flour in pancakes, muffins, and waffles. This is another highly absorbent Freebie Flour, so use ½ cup of flaxseed flour in place of 1 cup of flour.

ALMOND FLOUR. Almond flour is made from skinless, blanched almonds that have been finely ground. This Freebie Flour has a moist texture and rich, buttery flavor that makes great cakes and cookies. It can also be used to make crackers and chips. This flour is high in fiber, vitamin E, and magnesium. Magnesium has been shown to improve mood and reduce menopausal symptoms, and vitamin E has been shown to improve heart health.

For recipe ideas using these flours, visit JorgeCruise.com.

Trout

Tuna

Beef, Pork, Veal, Lamb

Bacon

Beef (trimmed of fat) including chuck, cubed, flank, porterhouse, rib, round, rump roast, sirloin, T-bone steak, tenderloin

Beef, ground

Beef jerky

Canadian bacon

Ham

Lamb chop, leg, or roast

Pork center loin chop

Pork tenderloin

Veal loin chop or roast

Other Proteins

Bierwurst or beerwurst

Bologna

Buffalo

Capicola

Chorizo

Corned beef

Devon (sausage)

Duck

Goose

Hot dog

Jay Robb Whey Protein

Liverwurst

Meatloaf

Pastrami

Pepperoni

Pheasant (no skin)

Pork roll

Processed sandwich/deli meats: chicken, ham, roast beef, turkey, etc.

Prosciutto

Salami

Sausage

Smoked meat

Summer sausage

Vegetarian Meats

Chik'n Strips: MorningStar Farms Meal Starters

Hot dogs: Lightlife Smart Dogs

Tofu

Veggie burgers: MorningStar Farms Garden Veggie Patties

VEGETABLES
—0 SUGAR CALORIES

Alfalfa sprouts

Artichokes

Arugula

Asparagus

Bell pepper, red

Bok choy, regular or baby

Broccoli

Brussels sprouts

Cabbage

Cauliflower

Celery

Chard, Swiss

Collards

Corn, white

Cucumber

Eggplant

Endive

Fennel

Green onion

Kale

Lettuce, iceberg

Lettuce, red leaf

Lettuce, romaine

Mushrooms

Mustard greens

Okra

Pepper, jalapeño

Pepper, serrano

Pickles, dill

Radicchio

Radishes

Scallions

Seaweed

Shallots

Snap peas

Spinach

Summer squash

Turnip greens

Watercress

Zucchini

HERBS & SPICES
—0 SUGAR CALORIES

Basil, fresh

Chives

Cilantro

Garlic

Ginger

Oregano

Parsley

Pepper

Peppermint, fresh

Salt

Thyme, fresh

FATS
—0 SUGAR CALORIES

Animal fats

Avocado oil

Barlean's Coconut Oil

Barlean's Flaxseed Oil

Butter

Ghee

Olive oil

Saturated fats

Sesame oil

Walnut oil

DAIRY PRODUCTS
—0 SUGAR CALORIES

Cheese

American

Asiago

Blue

Brick

Brie

Cheddar

Colby

Colby Jack

Cottage cheese

Cream cheese

Dry Jack

Edam

Farmer cheese

Feta

Fontina

STRIVE FOR **SAMENESS**

Try to eat the same way every day. A British study found that women who ate the same number of meals each day at the same time ate less food than those who didn't. Foods that keep you feeling full longer make it easier to stay consistent. Curb cravings with foods like low-fat yogurt and fresh fruit, a hard-cooked egg with whole-grain toast, or peanut butter on celery sticks.

Gorgonzola

Gouda

Gruyère

Havarti

Limburger

Mascarpone

Monterey Jack

Mozzarella

Muenster

Parmesan

Pepato

Pepper Jack

Provolone

Queso Blanco

Ricotta

Romano

Scamorza

String cheese

Soy cheese

Swiss

Teleme

Other Dairy and Dairy Alternatives

Almond milk, unsweetened

Coconut milk, unsweetened

FAGE Total Greek Yogurt

Half-and-half

Sour cream

Soy milk, unsweetened

Whipped cream

_____

OTHER AMAZING FREEBIES
—0 SUGAR CALORIES

Almonds

Almond butter, unsweetened

Almond flour/meal

Avocado

Balsamic vinegar

Baking powder

Baking soda

Barlean's Forti-Flax

Blue cheese dressing

Brazil nuts

Cashews

Chia flour

Coconut flour

Coconut, unsweetened flakes, shreds

Coffee, black

Espresso

Flax meal/flour

Hot sauce

Italian dressing

Lemon

Lime

Macadamia nuts

Mayonnaise

Mustard

Onion

Pecans

Pine nuts

Powdered mix, Stevita Tropical Singles

Pumpkin seeds

Ranch dressing

Salsa

Sesame seeds

Soy sauce

Sparkling water

Stevia

Sunflower seeds

Tea, unsweetened plain, hot or iced

Tomato

Truvia

Vinegar

Walnuts

Water

SUGAR CALORIE FOODS

Here's a list of many common foods that you must count toward your daily allowance of 100 Sugar Calories. If a food is not listed below but is not on the Freebie list, look up the Total Carbohydrate amount and multiply by 4 to get the Sugar Calorie total.

DAIRY PRODUCTS

Milk, 1% or fat free (1 cup) =
49 Sugar Calories

Milk, whole (1 cup) =
51 Sugar Calories

Nonfat dry milk (⅓ cup) =
12 Sugar Calories

Rice milk, plain, Rice Dream (1 cup) =
92 Sugar Calories

Soy milk, plain, Silk (1 cup) =
32 Sugar Calories

Yogurt, fat-free plain (6 ounces) =
52 Sugar Calories

LEGUMES

Black beans, cooked (½ cup) =
92 Sugar Calories

Baked beans, original, Bush Brothers (¼ cup) =
116 Sugar Calories

Chickpeas/garbanzo beans (½ cup) =
65 Sugar Calories

Edamame shelled soybeans (½ cup) =
40 Sugar Calories

Green beans (1 cup) =
32 Sugar Calories

Hummus (2 tablespoons) =
16 Sugar Calories

Kidney beans (¼ cup) =
40 Sugar Calories

Lentils (¼ cup) =
40 Sugar Calories

Pinto beans (¼ cup) =
44 Sugar Calories

BREADS AND TORTILLAS

Bagels, honey whole wheat (1) =
224 Sugar Calories

Bread, sprouted whole grain (1 slice) =
60 Sugar Calories

Bread, whole wheat (1 slice) =
88 Sugar Calories

Hamburger bun (1) =
72 Sugar Calories

Hamburger bun, sprouted whole grain (1) =
136 Sugar Calories

Pancakes, plain frozen, ready-to-heat (4″ diameter, 1) =
60 Sugar Calories

Pita, whole wheat (1) =
62 Sugar Calories

Roll, small dinner (1) =
52 Sugar Calories

Tortilla, corn (6″ diameter, 1) =
23 Sugar Calories

Tortilla, flour (6″ diameter, 1) =
64 Sugar Calories

Wrap, organic whole wheat (1) =
80 Sugar Calories

Waffles, frozen, ready-to-heat (4″ diameter, 1) =
60 Sugar Calories

PASTA

Penne, whole wheat, cooked (1 cup) =
208 Sugar Calories

Spaghetti, whole wheat, cooked (1 cup) =
151 Sugar Calories

Spirals, whole wheat, cooked (1 cup) =
149 Sugar Calories

CEREALS AND GRAINS

Basmati rice, cooked (½ cup) =
88 Sugar Calories

Brown rice, cooked (½ cup) =
92 Sugar Calories

Cereal, dry, Cheerios (¾ cup) =
72 Sugar Calories

Cereal, dry, Post Shredded Wheat (1 cup) =
164 Sugar Calories

Cereal, dry, Total (¾ cup) =
92 Sugar Calories

Cereal, dry, Uncle Sam's (¾ cup) =
152 Sugar Calories

Cereal, dry, Wheaties (¾ cup) =
88 Sugar Calories

Cereal, dry, whole grain ground flax, Ezekiel 4:9 (¾ cup) =
222 Sugar Calories

Cereal, dry, whole grain, Ezekiel 4:9 (½ cup) =
160 Sugar Calories

Corn muffin mix, Jiffy (¼ cup) =
108 Sugar Calories

Couscous, cooked (½ cup) =
73 Sugar Calories

Granola, low-fat (½ cup) =
160 Sugar Calories

Jasmine rice, cooked (½ cup) =
106 Sugar Calories

Oatmeal, dry steel-cut (¼ cup) =
108 Sugar Calories

Oatmeal, Quaker Instant Apples and Cinnamon (1 packet) =
88 Sugar Calories

Oatmeal, Quaker Original Instant (1 packet) =
76 Sugar Calories

Quinoa, cooked (½ cup) =
79 Sugar Calories

Spanish rice, cooked (½ cup) =
80 Sugar Calories

White rice, cooked (½ cup) =
106 Sugar Calories

VEGETABLES

Corn, yellow (½ cup) =
58 Sugar Calories

French fries, fast-food (1 large) =
260 Sugar Calories

Potato (1 medium) =
146 Sugar Calories

Rutabaga, cubes (1 cup) =
58 Sugar Calories

Sweet potato (1 medium) =
92 Sugar Calories

Turnip, cubes (1 cup) =
34 Sugar Calories

Vegetable blend, stir-fry, frozen (¾ cup) =
20 Sugar Calories

Winter squash, acorn (½ cup) =
75 Sugar Calories

Winter squash, butternut (½ cup) =
43 Sugar Calories

Yam (½ cup) =
75 Sugar Calories

FRUITS

A note about fruits: Fruits are healthy and have lots of vitamins—but they are primarily carbohydrates and natural sugar, so we do need to pay attention to calories because they spike insulin. The jury is out on these foods. Some agencies and experts say that the sugar and carbs in fruit shouldn't count because they're offset by fiber and water content, but others say that it can still alter weight loss. Based on this, I suggest keeping fruit servings to no more than two a day.

Apple (1 medium) =
99 Sugar Calories

Apricot (1 medium) =
16 Sugar Calories

Banana (1 medium) =
108 Sugar Calories

Blackberries (½ cup) =
29 Sugar Calories

Blueberries (½ cup) =
43 Sugar Calories

Cantaloupe (1 wedge) =
19 Sugar Calories

Cherries (9) =
47 Sugar Calories

Cherry tomatoes (½ cup) =
12 Sugar Calories

Dried bananas (¼ cup) =
240 Sugar Calories

Honeydew (1 wedge) =
46 Sugar Calories

Kiwi (1 medium) =
40 Sugar Calories

Mango, sliced (½ cup) =
52 Sugar Calories

Oranges (1 small) =
45 Sugar Calories

Peach (1 medium) =
59 Sugar Calories

Pear (1 small) =
92 Sugar Calories

Pineapple, diced (½ cup) =
43 Sugar Calories

Plum (1 medium) =
30 Sugar Calories

Plum tomatoes (½ cup) =
20 Sugar Calories

Raspberries (1 cup) =
59 Sugar Calories

Red and pink grapefruit (½) =
21 Sugar Calories

Tangerines (1 medium) =
47 Sugar Calories

Watermelon, diced (1 cup) =
46 Sugar Calories

SNACKS & TREATS

Cheese puffs, Cheetos Jumbo (1 ounce) =
60 Sugar Calories

Chips, Doritos Nacho Cheese (1 ounce) =
68 Sugar Calories

Chips, Kettle Lightly Salted (1 ounce) =
76 Sugar Calories

Chips, Popchips Original (22 chips) =
80 Sugar Calories

Chocolate, Green and Black's Organic Dark 85% (12 pieces) =
60 Sugar Calories

Cookies, Joseph's Chocolate Chip or Oatmeal (4 cookies) =
52 Sugar Calories

Cookies, Newman's Own Chocolate Crème (2 cookies) =
80 Sugar Calories

Corn snack, Pirate's
Booty (1 ounce) =
72 Sugar Calories

Crackers, Nabisco
Ritz Original (5) =
40 Sugar Calories

Crackers, Nabisco Wheat
Thins Multi-Grain (6) =
88 Sugar Calories

Crackers, Pepperidge Farms
Goldfish (55 pieces) =
80 Sugar Calories

Crispbread, Wasa
Original (2 pieces) =
80 Sugar Calories

Granola bars, oats,
fruits & nuts (1 bar) =
88 Sugar Calories

Ice cream, soft-serve,
vanilla (½ cup) =
70 Sugar Calories

Kettle corn (1 cup) =
100 Sugar Calories

Popcorn, air-popped
(3 cups) =
75 Sugar Calories

Rice cakes, Quaker Lightly
Salted (2) =
56 Sugar Calories

Trail mix (1 ounce) =
45 Sugar Calories

BEVERAGES

Apple juice (8 ounces) =
116 Sugar Calories

Beer, Coors Light
(1 bottle) =
20 Sugar Calories

LET'S TALK ABOUT **ALCOHOL**

My basic advice: Avoid alcohol. But, I'm also a realist. There'll be times when you'll want to have a drink (or two)—celebrations, happy hours, work events, holidays. So, let me give you some advice if you plan to indulge: Drink intelligently so your carb consumption is minimal. Here are some ideas.

- Drink low-carb beers: Michelob Ultra, Budweiser Select 55, Miller 64, and Rolling Rock Light all come in at around 2.5 grams of carbs or less per bottle.

- Ordering a cocktail? Have something sophisticated on the rocks instead of something sweet and frozen. Slushy fruit drinks tend to be made with bottled mixers that contain added sugar and syrups.

- Nurse a single glass of wine instead of drinking two beers.

- Sip a glass of water between drinks. This will help fill you and keep you away from hors d'oeuvres cravings. Plus, pacing yourself will cut back on the amount of alcohol you drink.

- If you ever find that you have difficulty stopping after a maximum of two drinks, avoid alcohol.

Beer, Michelob Ultra
(1 bottle) =
10 Sugar Calories

Beer, Miller Lite
(1 bottle) =
13 Sugar Calories

Beer, O'Doul's
Nonalcoholic (1 bottle) =
53 Sugar Calories

Cola, Diet Coke (8 ounces) =
*0 Sugar Calories (contains
artificial sweeteners)*

Energy drink, diet,
Rockstar (8 ounces) =
*8 Sugar Calories (contains
artificial sweeteners)*

Energy drink,
sugar-free, Red Bull
(8 ounces) =
*11 Sugar Calories (contains
artificial sweeteners)*

Ginger ale, Schweppes
(4 ounces) =
46 Sugar Calories

Grapefruit juice,
Ocean Spray Light
(8 ounces) =
120 Sugar Calories

Soda, Steaz Organic
Sparkling Green Tea
(1 can) =
92 Sugar Calories

Sports drink,
Gatorade Lemonade
(4 ounces) =
30 Sugar Calories

Vegetable juice,
V8 100% (8 ounces) =
40 Sugar Calories

Wine, dessert
(1 glass, 3 ounces) =
80 Sugar Calories

Wine, red
(1 glass, 3 ounces) =
14 Sugar Calories

Wine, white
(1 glass, 3 ounces) =
15 Sugar Calories

―――――――――――――

CONDIMENTS & DRESSINGS

Apple sauce, unsweetened
(½ cup) =
56 Sugar Calories

Barbecue sauce
(2 tablespoons) =
102 Sugar Calories

Cocktail sauce (⅛ cup) =
30 Sugar Calories

Honey (1 tablespoon) =
69 Sugar Calories

Ketchup (1 tablespoon) =
15 Sugar Calories

Miracle Whip, light
(2 tablespoons) =
24 Sugar Calories

Natural sweetener,
Xylitol Crystals
(1 tablespoon) =
24 Sugar Calories

Peanut butter
(2 tablespoons) =
25 Sugar Calories

Ranch dressing
(2 tablespoons) =
8 Sugar Calories

Teriyaki, ready-to-serve
(2 tablespoons) =
28 Sugar Calories

―――――――――――――

FROZEN FOODS
Amy's Frozen Meals

Black Bean and
Vegetable Enchilada =
88 Sugar Calories

Mexican Tofu
Scramble =
160 Sugar Calories

Shepherd's Pie =
108 Sugar Calories

Spinach Feta Pocket
Sandwich =
136 Sugar Calories

Lean Cuisine Frozen Meals

Alfredo Pasta with
Chicken & Broccoli =
180 Sugar Calories

Baked Chicken =
120 Sugar Calories

Beef Pot Roast =
104 Sugar Calories

Chicken and Vegetables =
116 Sugar Calories

Chicken Marsala =
116 Sugar Calories

Garlic Beef and Broccoli =
172 Sugar Calories

Grilled Chicken
Caesar Bowl =
132 Sugar Calories

Lemongrass Chicken =
140 Sugar Calories

Meatloaf with Gravy &
Whipped Potatoes =
100 Sugar Calories

Roasted Chicken with
Lemon Pepper Fettuccini =
112 Sugar Calories

Roasted Garlic Chicken =
44 Sugar Calories

Roasted Turkey
& Vegetables =
72 Sugar Calories

Rosemary Chicken =
108 Sugar Calories

Salmon with Basil =
100 Sugar Calories

Salisbury Steak
with Mac & Cheese =
92 Sugar Calories

Shrimp Alfredo =
112 Sugar Calories

Shrimp and Angel
Hair Pasta =
136 Sugar Calories

Steak Tips Portobello =
56 Sugar Calories

Stuffed Cabbage =
112 Sugar Calories

Swedish Meatballs =
140 Sugar Calories

FOODS TO AVOID!

As I've said, not all carbs are bad. But many are. I won't flat-out say, "Avoid these foods at all costs!" (You may have seen some of them on the previous lists.) But I will advise you to avoid them *whenever you can.* The reason is so simple: If you stay away from them, losing weight will be easier. That's a good enough reason for anyone, right?

"White" foods

White bread

White flour pitas

White flour products,
like baked goods

White pasta

White rice

Sweeteners

Agave syrup

Corn syrup

Flavored coffee creamers
and additives

High fructose corn syrup

Honey

Maple syrup

Molasses

Processed sugar

Sucrose

Table syrup

Artificial sweeteners

Equal

Splenda

Sweet'N Low

Beverages

Alcohol
(see "Let's Talk About
Alcohol" on page 177)

Diet soda

Energy drinks, like Red Bull

Fruit juices
(eat a piece of whole
fruit instead)

Kool-Aid and similar
"fruit drinks"

Lemonade

Soda

Sweetened tea

Breakfast foods

Cereal bars

French toast

Hash browns or
fried potatoes

Pancakes

Processed breakfast
shakes

Sweetened cereals

Toaster pastries

Waffles

Snacks and Sides

Breaded foods
(this goes for entrées, too)

Fried foods
(this goes for entrées, too)

French fries

Potato chips and other
bagged snack chips

Pretzels

Non-wheat-based
crackers

Desserts

Cake

Cookies

Brownies

Ice cream/frozen yogurt

Pie (even with whole fruit)

DON'T FORGET ABOUT **SALT!**

I talk an awful lot about carbs, but I also want you to remember to watch your sodium intake. Salt is terrific as a seasoning when used sparingly. But many foods—especially processed foods, cold cuts, and restaurant meals—are packed with salt. Too much salt in your diet can lead to unwanted consequences like high blood pressure and water retention. Preparing your own meals is the best way to control your salt intake. After all, if you make it, you know exactly what's in it. A good motto: When a recipe says "salt to taste" that doesn't mean "salt to death!"

Candy

It may seem obvious to say avoid candy of any kind because the major ingredient is sugar. But sweets come in many forms, and some can be worse for you than others. Why? Because they're deceptive. Many come in shapes and sizes that tempt you to eat more. For example, you know that you should avoid candy bars—and it's easy to stop after one. However, it's not as easy to stop eating candy that comes in a bag or box (or know exactly how much you're eating). Here are some examples.

Candy corn

Chocolate-covered anything

Chocolates/bonbons

Fudge

Hard candy

M&M's

Mini versions of candy bars

Reese's Pieces

Skittles

Swedish Fish

Tootsie Rolls

Chapter
7

Inches
Off! Your
Tummy:
Week 5
and
Beyond

"It's always too early to quit."

—NORMAN VINCENT PEALE

Congratulations! You've made it through the first 4 weeks of Inches Off! Your Tummy—so now what? On the following pages you'll find suggestions for how to keep the Inches Off! workouts going and stay on track. I will address how to deal with cravings and overcome motivational challenges, so you don't get sidelined from your goals!

WHERE DOES THE 5-MINUTE FITNESS FORMULA GO FROM HERE?

You can easily continue my program by simply repeating the 4 weeks over again. Or you can create your own 5-minute plan by mixing and matching the days in the planner from Chapter 3. Just make sure to get the workouts you'll be doing in your planner—I suggest writing down a week's worth on your Sunday rest day, so you won't have to think about what you'll be doing on a day-to-day basis when schedules can get busy.

Make copies of the blank planner on pages 184–185 and then write in the workouts you'll be doing as well as the page numbers for the exercise descriptions. It will work as an easy reference for you all week long.

CRUSH CRAVINGS AND STOP SELF-SABOTAGE!

As the weeks move forward, some people find that their motivation wavers and cravings become harder to ignore. Be aware of your weak spots and read the following to bolster your resolve.

We all have a weak spot.

You know what I mean: It's that place where your willpower wilts and you eat something you shouldn't. I'm talking about a literal spot, a physical place in your home where you stand and make a bad decision.

For some, it's right in front of the fridge. For others, it's over near the countertop

(continued on page 186)

IDENTIFY **YOUR WEAK SPOTS**

A weak spot is an actual location—a place where you always seem to make a poor lifestyle choice. Take a minute and write down these locations in your life: the fridge, a candy drawer, a bar, or a drive-thru. Make a master list of all the places that put you in a weakened position when it comes to eating or drinking something you know you shouldn't.

At first, avoiding these weak spots will help you stay on track for weight loss and fitness success. But later, as you understand the emotional response these places bring out in you, you won't have to avoid them. You'll know how to manage your feelings at their core.

Week 5 and beyond

(Exercise descriptions start on page 36).

WORKOUT
WEEKS

5

and
Beyond . . .

Day 1	Day 2	Day 3
60 SECONDS: (exercise name)	**60 SECONDS:** (exercise name)	**60 SECONDS:** (exercise name)
60 SECONDS: (exercise name)	**60 SECONDS:** (exercise name)	**60 SECONDS:** (exercise name)
60 SECONDS: (exercise name)	**60 SECONDS:** (exercise name)	**60 SECONDS:** (exercise name)
60 SECONDS: (exercise name)	**60 SECONDS:** (exercise name)	**60 SECONDS:** (exercise name)
60 SECONDS: (exercise name)	**60 SECONDS:** (exercise name)	**60 SECONDS:** (exercise name)

Day 4	Day 5	Day 6	Day 7
60 SECONDS: (exercise name) _____ _____	**60 SECONDS:** (exercise name) _____ _____	**60 SECONDS:** (exercise name) _____ _____	Rest day. Enjoy a family bike ride, walk your dog, or take a swim.
60 SECONDS: (exercise name) _____ _____	**60 SECONDS:** (exercise name) _____ _____	**60 SECONDS:** (exercise name) _____ _____	
60 SECONDS: (exercise name) _____ _____	**60 SECONDS:** (exercise name) _____ _____	**60 SECONDS:** (exercise name) _____ _____	
60 SECONDS: (exercise name) _____ _____	**60 SECONDS:** (exercise name) _____ _____	**60 SECONDS:** (exercise name) _____ _____	
60 SECONDS: (exercise name) _____ _____	**60 SECONDS:** (exercise name) _____ _____	**60 SECONDS:** (exercise name) _____ _____	

If you find that the exercises are feeling too easy, increase the weight of the dumbbell, resistance band, or medicine ball you are using. If you desire a longer workout, you can repeat the routine twice for a 10-minute burn.

next to the coffeemaker, where the cookie jar is or the plate of cupcakes sits. Maybe you prefer the pantry and its chip bags. Or the second shelf in the freezer, where the ice cream calls to you like some kind of supernatural force.

Oh, and let's not forget the supposedly healthy spots. The dinner table, where a second or third helping of protein and an indulgent starch seem okay—even though you know you're already full. Or the drawer in your office or cubicle, where you have your mixed nuts stashed . . . and you're restocking that drawer a lot more than you should (and you know it). Too much of a good thing can be bad, after all.

You can have a weak spot outside of home and work, too. A bar where you meet coworkers or friends. A candy shop on the corner. The coffee shop where you buy your daily 20-ounce, 5-dollar, 600-calorie pick-me-up. The drive-thru on the way home.

Oh yeah, you know exactly what I'm talking about.

So where are your weak spots?

Here's the thing: There is nothing evil about these spots. They're just . . . there. But they've come to mean something to you *on an emotional level.*

That's the problem. A very fixable problem.

STAY ON TOP OF
YOUR EMOTIONS

One of the ways you can make sure to stay on track toward your goals is to be in touch with your emotions. Emotions lie at the core of any health and fitness plan. The gym, the exercise gear, the workout clothes—all these things are just window dressing. Real results come from your

---

WORDPLAY!

Don't let certain words undermine your emotions and motivation. See how simple word choices can change how you think.

- **You don't want to be "thin" or "skinny."** These can be negative descriptions associated with unhealthy eating, fad dieting, and the media and Hollywood.

- **You want to be "lean" and "healthy."** These are *always* positive outcomes. Who doesn't want to be lean and healthy!?

See how something as simple as word choice can alter your outlook?

emotional core. Why? Our emotions, more than anything, rule our decision-making process. Do any of the following sound familiar?

- **ENVY.** Why can't I look like the slim, fit people I see all around me?

- **ANGER.** Why did life deal me these cards? Why is losing weight and exercising so hard for me?

- **GUILT.** Why didn't I exercise today? Why did I eat the whole thing?

- **SELF-DEFEAT.** I can't do it. It's too hard.

- **SELF-LOATHING.** I hate my body. I hate my life.

Any of these feelings and thought patterns will directly affect your decision making. That's why it's so crucial to understand your emotional responses, which can lead to emotional eating and skipping exercise. Understand them and you'll find it much easier to release yourself from all the willpower battles, depressing internal monologues, and self-inflicted guilt trips about failure.

HOW TO SOLVE
EMOTIONAL EATING

Many people can easily follow the simple nutrition ideas in this book and never feel tempted to overeat. But I know that some of you need a little extra help—particularly those of you who tend to eat for emotional, rather than physical, reasons.

What is emotional eating exactly? It happens anytime you eat to mask or numb a negative feeling. You do it when you're not hungry, and it's the number one thing that can cause self-sabotage. How important is this? Well, I feel that what I am about to share with you is the most important section of the book! Indeed, if you don't master this step, you will never achieve the results you want.

Emotions rank as the number one most powerful cause of overeating. Before they came to me for coaching, many of my clients used food as an emotional support for the distress in their lives. They lifted sadness with ice cream, covered up depression with chocolate chip cookies, and soothed anger with potato chips.

This is addictive behavior. I'm not suggesting that you're addicted to food. But if you consume unhealthy amounts of anything—food, alcohol, or drugs like nicotine or worse—to mask an emotional feeling, that's an addictive tendency.

Sure enough, when I explored the cause of my clients' emotional eating, I found that the true source of the problem stemmed from an emotional void or emptiness. They felt empty, and they filled up that emptiness with food.

Think about it. In the past, when you ate when you were not hungry, did food help fill a void or numb a pain? Has food ever made you feel supported and comforted?

Remember what I told you about my own weight and eating problems? I felt like an outcast as a kid. When I got home every day, the love of my family—in the form of *huge* meals—filled that hole in my heart. I was a classic emotional eater. But once I identified what brought that on, I was able to make better choices—almost instantly!

To stop the self-sabotage and end emotional eating, you must learn to discern between emotional hunger and nutritional hunger. **Nutritional, or body, hunger** is a biological need. It's all about eating to provide your body with the building materials it needs to stay healthy and create lean muscle.

Emotional, or mind, hunger often comes from lack of support, comfort, and warm nurturing from people. Only when you replace food with support from friends and family will you be able to step off the emotional-eating roller coaster.

So how do you beat such a powerful negative force in your life?

I have a tested-and-proven technique that I call the People Solution. It gives all my clients strong protection from emotional eating. Since I started using it, I've heard tons of success stories from readers who tried it and loved it. The People Solution teaches you how to replace the comfort of food with the support of people. It includes three key tactics.

1. Become your own best friend. The first person in The People Solution is you. Too often, people have a love-hate relationship with their bodies. (Remember all those negative emotional responses you just read about?) Yet you

---

THE MOTIVATOR CHANGE YOUR MIND.

A lot of people have strong beliefs. But don't ever let negative beliefs hold you back from doing the right thing for yourself. For example, if you've tried several diets before and have never been able to sustain success, you can start to believe that you're not destined to succeed. That's a fixed mind-set. With a fixed mind-set, you have a belief—maybe without even realizing it—that your qualities are carved in stone. And since any failure is a big verdict (you're a loser), you stick with what you know. And you never grow. So embrace a growth mind-set. It's easy. No matter what happens, simply ask yourself, "How can I learn from and use what just happened?"

must respect your body and treat it as the greatest gift you've ever received if you want to experience success. Only when you respect your body will you commit to transforming it.

To help make this happen, I suggest that all of my clients create what I call a Power Pledge Poster. On the poster they write the phrase, "My current body is the most precious gift I have ever been given." Underneath that, they write the positive consequences of believing that statement. For example, you might write, "I will treat my body as a top priority," or "I will feed my body properly." Then, underneath those consequences, write 10 sentences that describe why your body is a precious gift. For example, you might write, "My body helps me to get to where I need to go." I encourage you to create your own Power Pledge Poster. After you do so, photocopy it three times and post it in three spots in your house or at work where you will see it often.

2. Establish a support circle. This is the second set of people in the People Solution. I encourage all of my clients to create a support network of— at minimum—three people that will help motivate them to stick to their program. Your inner circle can include family, coworkers, church members, and, of course, your good friends. You should choose people that allow you to feel comfortable communicating your feelings. Some of these people should be e-mail buddies—people you can e-mail at any time of the day or night when you feel you might be about to slip up. Others might be phone buddies—people who will agree to literally be on call in case you need support. One person should be an accountability buddy—someone you can meet with once a week to go over the specifics of the program along with your challenges and breakthroughs.

3. Expand your circle. In addition to picking three people you already

CHOOSE **YOUR FRIENDS WISELY**

Some scary research: People tend to mirror the habits and attitudes of those closest to them. If your family and friends have negative attitudes, are overweight, or have lousy habits, you probably do, too. If the opposite is true, you're more likely to have good habits and a positive outlook.

In other words, *you are who you hang out with.*

This can force difficult choices. If you truly want to transform your body and life, you need to seek out loved ones who won't (consciously or unconsciously) encourage your self-sabotage.

LET'S TALK ABOUT **HAPPINESS**

You see the promises all the time: "If you just do this one thing, you'll be happy!" That one thing is whatever is being sold to you at that moment: a new pair of shoes, a car, a tech gadget, a restaurant, a cocktail, a movie, an expensive coffee, an expensive coffeemaker, a dating service, a . . . whatever. The message is everywhere, and it does not stop.

Have any of those things ever brought you lasting happiness? Of course not.

Here's why: Research shows that buying or acquiring a physical thing only brings fleeting bits of happiness. The euphoria you feel generally fades after a few weeks, at most, and usually sooner. Think about your own happiness purchases. That sounds about right, doesn't it?

Research also shows that the happiness you get from experiences, which produce memories, lasts much longer. Which is why, if you're determined to spend your money, a trip to somewhere you've never been will make you happier for a longer time than, say, a new iPad.

That's helpful information that I use myself. But you know what? When you're talking about long-lasting happiness—the stuff that really sticks—you have to go deeper.

I believe that happiness is a choice.

And usually it's a really, really difficult choice.

When you finally make the choice to have a happier life, those around you will be affected by it. And some may not like it at all. Here are some examples of what I mean.

- **You're overweight and choose to change your life.** You clean up your lifestyle, you start exercising, and you begin to look healthier . . . and all the people close to you who are still overweight and trapped in their bad habits resent you. They want you to look just like them.

- **You drink too much and choose to leave it behind.** If you're addicted, that will be difficult enough. But those around you—maybe your spouse, your best friend, or even everyone you know—belittle your sobriety. They want you to keep drinking with them.

- **You're in a long-term relationship that makes you unhappy every day.** You choose to get out, and maybe your significant other doesn't accept that you no longer want to share a life. They want you to stay because it's more about them than it is about you.

You see what I mean? Choosing happiness (or a chance at it) can be one of the most terrifying choices you'll ever make. It can literally change your entire life and the lives of your loved ones. It can even be seen as selfish by others.

I've had to make these choices myself. More than once. They were painful choices, but they were worth it. I'm happier now.

That's why I say happiness is a choice. Happiness takes guts. But if it's the right choice for you, you have to make it.

know to help support your efforts, you will continually add more people to your inner circle. You might do that by joining or starting a Jorge Cruise weight-loss book group, or by going online to jorgecruise.com or facebook.com/jorgecruisefan and meeting millions of Cruisers who are taking the same journey as you!

THE MOTIVATOR GO PUBLIC.

Tell people who will hold you accountable that you're dedicated to losing weight. They have permission to help you—in positive ways—stay on track. When people step in and tell you that "I believe in you" and "I'm going to help you," it encourages and motivates you and it gives you the freedom to make big changes.

"I couldn't wait for success so I went ahead without it."

—JONATHAN WINTERS

So far in this book, we've talked a lot about fitness and food. If you stick with the plan, you'll get terrific results. But what if I told you that you could do even better? That there are several smart and simple things you can do to help maximize the results you see? Wouldn't it be a no-brainer to do those things?

Well, here they are. I assembled them in one place to make it even easier for you. Think of these suggestions as nice little bonuses to the Inches Off! plan, but there's more to it than that. You see, this chapter isn't just about slimming your tummy or losing a set amount of goal weight. The things you read here are also about living a better life. I know from experience that if you use them, your day-to-day health and energy will be even stronger.

So what's not to like? Read on, and find out how to live better, one good habit at a time.

THE MAGIC POWER
OF SLEEP

Everyone knows that you're supposed to get 7 to 8 hours of sleep a night. It's not always easy, and we often will skimp on sleep and not feel bad about it. On the other hand, skipping a workout or eating a lavish meal is enough to trigger the guilts. But you're on the Inches Off! plan now, and here's something I never hear people talk about: Exercise and sleep go together like fish and water (or maybe fish, some olive oil, garlic, lemon, and a hot grill). How so?

A good night's sleep can help you have a stronger workout. And a stronger workout can improve your sleep quality. Plus, a majority of the good stuff from exercise—like muscles repairing themselves, bones strengthening— happens while you sleep. As important as exercise is, sleep is the most important activity of your day.

There are other reasons to take sleep more seriously. For example, sleep affects your diet. Think about it: When do you feel most in the mood for a greasy fast food meal or a big plate of comfort food? After a beautiful night's sleep? Or after 5 or 6 hours of lousy shut-eye? Exactly. Sleep deprivation can affect appetite and metabolism, leading to overeating and, over time, weight gain and obesity. Poor sleep can also raise your blood pressure and make you produce stress hormones like cortisol that signal your body to store belly fat. Chronic sleep deprivation is sneaky: It may feel so normal to you that you don't realize the damage you're causing, inside or outside, or how much your day-to-day effectiveness could improve if you got more sleep.

To give you a better idea of how beneficial regular sleep is, look at what happens through an average night . . .

There are four stages of sleep. The first two are transition phases from wakefulness and typically take just a few minutes each. During the third phase, deep sleep, your body releases growth hormone, builds new muscle, and repairs damages caused by stress. REM sleep, a lighter phase during which you dream, seems to improve learning and cognition. People learning new mental skills have trouble recalling them if deprived of this phase of sleep.

One pass through these four stages takes roughly 90 minutes, and the cycle repeats four to six times per night. The amount of time you spend in each phase shifts as the night goes on. Most people have more deep sleep at the beginning of the night and more REM sleep closer to morning. Staying up late, then, tends to deprive you of deep sleep, whereas rising early can cut down on REM time.

Anything less than 7 hours of sleep can affect you both physically and mentally. But the quality of sleep is often just as important as the quantity. Have you ever spent 7 to 9 hours in bed but not felt rested the next day? It's common for a lot of people, and it's usually due to one or a combination of the following factors . . .

- Sleep apnea, a condition where your breathing is

interrupted and you awaken multiple times through the night (sometimes without knowing it). Certain factors, from being overweight to head position, can obstruct your airways. Snoring is the big giveaway here.

- Stress and anxiety

- Loud noises, including crying children and loud neighbors

- Pain

- Late-night consumption of alcohol or caffeine

- GERD (gastroesophageal reflux disorder)

- Certain medicines, including steroids, beta-blockers, and pain medications

- The herbal supplements ginseng and guarana

I have a useful list of strategies I use to help my sleep quality. Give 'em a try. The first thing I do is hold my sleeping time sacred. I respect it. I understand that it's the only time I will have to make sure I'm at my best the next day.

10
Tips

1 SET A SLEEP SCHEDULE— AND STICK WITH IT

If you do only one thing to improve your sleep, this is it: Go to bed at the same time every night and get up at the same time every morning— even on weekends. A regular sleep routine keeps your biological clock steady so you rest better. Exposure to a regular pattern of light and dark helps, so stay in sync by opening the blinds or going outside right after you wake up.

2 CUT CAFFEINE AFTER 2 P.M.

In the morning, I love a fresh cup of coffee. The aroma and a bit of caffeine get me moving. However, having caffeine after 2 p.m. isn't recommended, because it stays in your system for 8 hours. So if you have black coffee after dinner, come bedtime, it'll either prevent your brain from entering deep sleep or stop you from falling asleep altogether.

3 TAKE TIME TO WIND DOWN

Give your body time to transition from your active day to bedtime drowsiness by setting a timer for an hour before bed. Use that time as follows:

• Prep for tomorrow (pack your bag, set out your clothes).

• Take care of personal hygiene (brush your teeth, moisturize your face).

• Relax in bed, reading with a small, low-wattage book light or practicing deep breathing.

I also like to stretch before bed. Basic yoga moves are nice, but keep reading for a set of in-bed stretches you can try (see pages 198–199).

4 BACK OFF THE BOOZE

A few hours after drinking, alcohol levels in your blood start to drop, which signals your body to wake up. It takes an average person about an hour to metabolize one drink, so if you have two glasses of wine with dinner, finish your last sip at least 2 hours before bed.

5 STAY COOL...

Experts usually recommend setting your bedroom thermostat between 65° and 75°F—a good guideline, but pay attention to how you actually feel under the covers. Slipping between cool sheets helps trigger a drop in your body temperature. That shift signals the body to produce melatonin, which induces sleep. That's why it's also a good idea to take a warm bath or hot shower before going to bed. Both temporarily raise your body temperature, after which it gradually lowers in the cooler air, cueing your body to feel sleepy.

6 ...ESPECIALLY IF YOU'RE MENOPAUSAL

During menopause, 75 percent of women suffer from hot flashes, and just over 20 percent have night sweats or hot flashes that interrupt their sleep. Consider turning on a fan or the AC to cool and circulate the air. Just go low gradually: Your body loses some ability to regulate its temperature during rapid eye movement (REM) sleep, so overchilling your environment— down to 60°F, for instance—will backfire.

7 TURN ON THE WHITE NOISE

Sound machines designed to help you sleep produce a low-level, soothing noise. These can help you tune out barking dogs, the TV downstairs, or any other disturbances so you can fall asleep and stay asleep.

8 ELIMINATE SNEAKY LIGHT SOURCES

Light tells your brain it's time to wake up. Even the glow from your laptop, iPad, smartphone, or any other electronics on your nightstand may pass through your closed eyelids and retinas into your hypothalamus, the part of your brain that controls sleep. This delays your brain's release of melatonin. Thus, the darker your room is, the more soundly you'll sleep.

9 CONSIDER KICKING OUT FURRY FRIENDS

If you own a cat, you already know how the little critters can be active in the late-night and early-morning hours. And dog owners know what kind of sniffing, grooming, and snoring noises they produce in a given night. More than half of people who sleep with their pets say the animals disturb their slumber, according to a survey from the Mayo Clinic Sleep Disorders Center. You may not like it, and your pet may really hate it, but if it means better sleep for you, don't let them in the bedroom at night.

10 STAY PUT IF YOU WAKE UP

Generally, if I wake up in the night and can't fall back asleep in 10 or 15 minutes, I stay in bed. I concentrate on deep breathing and stay relaxed, which usually works. I guess the real question to ask yourself is, "How do I feel?" If you're not fretting or anxious, I don't see a reason to get out of bed. But if lying in bed pushes your stress buttons, get up and do something quiet and relaxing, such as gentle yoga or massaging your feet until you feel sleepy again. Don't head for the kitchen for a midnight snack—it's too easy to overeat.

SLEEP BETTER WITH THESE STRETCHES

As I mentioned, some slow stretching or yoga before bed can be incredibly relaxing. Here are some stretches I do periodically, swapping in and out for variety.

STRETCH YOUR LOWER BACK

Lie on your back on the left side of your bed. Lift your right knee into your chest and then cross it over to the left side of your body. Let it hang slightly over the edge of the bed so gravity helps the stretch.

Extend your right arm in T position, palm facing down. Bring your left hand to your right hip and gently press your hip to the left to increase the stretch.

Turn your head to the right.

Hold for 30 seconds, then shift your body over to the right side of the bed and do this stretch with the left knee.

STRETCH YOUR GLUTE

Lie on your back with your legs extended. Slowly lift your right knee into your chest. Clasp your hands in front of your shin and gently pull your knee toward you to increase the stretch. Release any tension in your shoulders and neck. Keep your left leg relaxed in a comfortable position. Hold for 30 seconds and repeat with the left knee bent.

STRETCH YOUR HIPS

This stretch lengthens the lower back and opens up always-tight hips. Lie on your back with your legs extended. Lift your right knee and hold on to the sole of your foot with both hands. Press your knee down toward the bed so it's next to your torso, just below your shoulder. Your back and head should remain flat on the bed. Keep your left leg relaxed in a comfortable position. Hold for 30 seconds and then repeat with the left leg.

STRETCH YOUR QUAD

Lie on your left side with your head propped up by your left hand. Bend your right knee so your foot goes back toward your buttock. Grasp the top of your right foot with your right hand and pull your heel toward your buttock. Hold for 30 seconds, pressing your hips slightly forward to increase the stretch in the front of your thigh. Release the stretch, roll over onto your right side, and stretch your left quad.

STRETCH YOUR CORE

Roll over onto your belly and extend your arms out in front of you. Without lifting your pelvis or legs off the bed, walk your hands toward your chest. As your torso lifts off the bed, keep a slight bend in your elbows. Walk your hands in until you feel a nice stretch in your abs. Lift your head back between your shoulder blades, and you'll feel a nice stretch in your chest and neck.

Hold for 30 seconds and lower your torso back to the bed.

STRETCH YOUR SHOULDERS

Sit in the middle of your bed with your back straight and your legs extended in front of you. Lower your torso back so that your head is hanging off the bed. Extend your arms over your head and down to the floor. Relax your body. Let gravity help you deepen the stretch. Hold this position for 30 seconds, then bend your knees and put your hands behind your head to sit up.

Wake Up Like a Champion

As important as sleep is, I have some quick morning routines that get me out of bed with energy and a smile instead of wanting to hit the snooze button (everyone has days like that, but really, who has time?). If you get into the habit of both sleeping and waking up well, you might even eventually call yourself a morning person.

Drink instant energy. No, I don't mean sugary orange juice. Drinking a big glass of water as soon as you get up is a good way to replenish the fluid your body loses overnight, and it provides instant energy. Think about it: Everything that happens in your body requires water, and you just spent the last 8 hours slowly losing fluids from respiration and evaporation (and if your room is too warm, perspiration). Even a 2 percent drop in your body's water stores can tire you physically and mentally.

Let the sun hit you. You are not a vampire. When you get up, open a shade. Check news or morning e-mails by a sunny window or step outside for a few minutes while having that morning glass of water (or black coffee). Daylight signals your biological clock to stop the secretion of melatonin, a hormone that makes you sleepy, and tells you it's time to be awake. It also increases the brain's level of serotonin, a chemical that boosts mood. If it's still dark when you wake up, you can buy dawn simulators that gradually increase the light in your room on a timer. At the very least, you can switch on a lamp.

Breathe. Few of us breathe deeply or consciously. This is especially effective in the morning, filling your lungs and letting the oxygen bring you to life. Think about it: When was the last time you took a long, slow, deep breath and slowly let it out again? Deep breaths oxygenate your brain and tissues and help reduce stress hormones. Now have a shower—you have things to do!

HOW TO EAT SMART
WHEN YOU EAT OUT

Making a home-cooked meal is the easiest way to ensure better nutrition. You buy the ingredients and know exactly what goes into your meals. Unfortunately, some people don't have the time or confidence to cook on a daily basis. Some people, because of their careers, are traveling and eating out more often than they eat at home. In fact, the number of calories that Americans consume outside of their homes has doubled since the late 1970s—and that number is directly linked to our increase in weight gain.

Hey, I know—eating out can be amazing. You *want* it to be a nice experience. But be smart about it. Here are some tips for navigating a restaurant menu, so that you can lose weight without losing your favorite place to eat.

Control Your Environment

When you eat out, no one is going to control calories for you, and you shouldn't be expected to count calories for yourself. But these are the facts: You are likely to eat 36 percent more calories when you eat out than when you're at home. So you need to take steps that help limit your overindulgence.

Tip #1: Ask your server to remove the bread basket from the table. Bread is virtually all sugar calories.

Tip #2: Tell your server what you would like on your plate. If your meal comes with french fries or chips, ask for those to be left off your plate.

Tip #3: Ask for sauces or salad dressing to be brought on the side. This way you can add them in the amounts you need (not in the excess amounts that most restaurants provide).

Tip #4: It's very hard to overeat vegetables, but rice, potatoes, pastas, and breads are carbohydrate- and calorie-dense foods that can sabotage your weight loss. Order green!

Tip #5: When you order, ask for a spare plate. When your food comes, cut your portions in half and transfer half to the spare plate. Then ask your server to pack that food to go. You eat half the calories (and trust me, in most restaurants, that's plenty) and you have lunch for the following day. Two meals for the price of one!

PRETEND IT'S **1950**

There's a reason that people were slimmer back in the day. It's estimated that in the past 25 years, laborsaving devices have decreased the number of calories we burn by 800 per day. If you go by the old wisdom that says 3,500 calories equals a pound, that's about 1.5 pounds per week. Think of the possibilities—and energy burned—if you made a few little changes to take you back in time . . .

- Disconnect your garage door opener and do it by hand.

- Get up and change the channel without a remote.

- Ignore all drive-thrus. Park and walk inside.

- Instead of e-mailing a coworker, walk to her office.

- Walk somewhere you normally drive.

- Wash your car by hand.

- Leave your phone on a table across the room, as if it has a cord, and get up to answer it. Stand and pace while talking.

APPENDIX

Your Inches Off! 4-Week Day-By-Day Food Log

"What would life be if we had no courage to attempt anything?"

—VINCENT VAN GOGH

I've designed this book to be as user-friendly as possible. If you take a look at the workout section of this book, you can see—right on the page—what exercises you'll be doing each day and how to do them. Well, I wanted you to have the very same day-to-day information at your fingertips when it comes to eating.

People are different in what they want from an eating plan. Some people like to be given all the information they need for every meal so that all they have to do is cook it up. Some will use the given information as a set of suggestions and mix and match meals and snacks depending on what they want to eat from one day to the next. Other people like to take a blank page and fill it themselves with different food combinations from the Chapter 6 food lists or food ideas they find elsewhere.

I'm offering all those options!

In this special section, your daily log, you'll see prefilled suggestions for the following:

- Breakfast
- Morning snack
- Lunch
- Afternoon snack
- Dinner
- Dessert

With each food entry, you'll see how many Sugar Calories are in each food—or if the food is a Freebie. I'm only making suggestions, of course. Feel free to swap out, say, pumpkin seeds as a snack if you'd rather have almonds or string cheese. The plan is simple to follow, and if you do indeed follow it, you'll keep yourself well within the 100 Sugar Calories limit every single day. In fact, most days you'll hardly eat any Sugar Calories at all.

These daily logs contain other information as well. You'll be able to check off an exercise box to ensure you don't skip a workout. You'll also keep track of how much water you drink each day. Don't underestimate water. Your body runs on it. Even slight dehydration can lower your mental and physical performance during the day. So drink up!

I also want you to keep track of two other key factors: your sleep quality and your energy level. As you work through the 4-week program, you'll be able to identify patterns in sleep and energy. (If you're skimping on the shut-eye, for example, you'll be able to catalog how it affects you so you'll know what changes you need to make.)

What if you prefer to make up your own daily menus? Go for it! But I still suggest you keep a daily log that includes the "smaller" things like how much water you drink. Research has shown time and again that people who keep close track of everything they eat and drink have better weight-loss results. It's not hard to see why: You'll know exactly where you are, food-wise, every moment of the day. That leads to a very simple result: You'll never eat badly.

And if you never eat badly, you'll always be successful!

You can find blank log sheets to print out at JorgeCruise.com.

Happy eating!

YOUR INCHES OFF! DAILY LOG

MEAL: Breakfast	SUGAR CALORIES (carb grams x 4)
2 poached eggs	Freebie
½ cup spinach	Freebie
2 strips turkey bacon	Freebie
MEAL: Snack	
¼ cup pumpkin seeds	Freebie
MEAL: Lunch (toss the ingredients with salt and pepper to taste)	
½ cup steamed chopped cauliflower	Freebie
½ cup steamed chopped broccoli	Freebie
2 tablespoons chopped red bell pepper	Freebie
3 slices chopped ham	Freebie
2 tablespoons olive oil	Freebie
MEAL: Snack	
1 hard-cooked egg	Freebie
MEAL: Dinner	
3 ounces sliced cooked chicken breast	Freebie
2 cups mixed greens	Freebie
Olive oil and vinegar dressing	Freebie
Salt and pepper	Freebie
MEAL: Dessert	
1 (5-ounce) glass red wine	14
DAILY TOTAL	**14 Sugar Calories**

MY WATER INTAKE
(8-ounce glasses):

1 2 3 4 5 6 7 8 More?

MY SLEEP QUALITY LAST NIGHT
(10 is highest):

1 2 3 4 5 6 7 8 9 10

MY ENERGY LEVEL YESTERDAY
(10 is highest):

1 2 3 4 5 6 7 8 9 10

☐ YOUR **WORKOUT**

SQUAT AND PRESS
(x 3 minutes)

HIGH KNEES
(x 2 minutes)

YOUR INCHES OFF! DAILY LOG

MEAL: Breakfast	SUGAR CALORIES (carb grams x 4)
½ cup cottage cheese	Freebie
2 tablespoons chopped pecans	Freebie
Coffee with half-and-half	Freebie
MEAL: Snack	
1 stick string cheese	Freebie
MEAL: Lunch (toss the ingredients together)	
5 medium shrimp	Freebie
2 cups shredded romaine	Freebie
5 cherry tomatoes	Freebie
2 tablespoons Caesar dressing	4
MEAL: Snack	
5 celery sticks spread with cream cheese	Freebie
MEAL: Dinner (prepare as an open-faced burger)	
1 slice Food For Life Ezekiel 4:9 Sprouted Grain Bread	60
1 slice provolone	Freebie
3 ounces cooked lean ground beef patty	Freebie
1 tablespoon mustard	Freebie
¼ cup arugula	Freebie
MEAL: Dessert	
1 (5-ounce) glass red wine	14
DAILY TOTAL	**78 Sugar Calories**

☐ YOUR **WORKOUT**

SUMO DEADLIFT HIGH PULL
(x 3 minutes)

PLANK
(x 2 minutes)

MY WATER INTAKE
(8-ounce glasses):
1 2 3 4 5 6 7 8 More?

MY SLEEP QUALITY LAST NIGHT
(10 is highest):
1 2 3 4 5 6 7 8 9 10

MY ENERGY LEVEL YESTERDAY
(10 is highest):
1 2 3 4 5 6 7 8 9 10

205

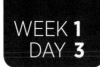

WEEK 1
DAY 3

YOUR INCHES OFF! DAILY LOG

MEAL: Breakfast	SUGAR CALORIES (carb grams x 4)
2 poached eggs	Freebie
½ cup spinach	Freebie
2 strips turkey bacon	Freebie
MEAL: Snack	
¼ cup pumpkin seeds	Freebie
MEAL: Lunch (mix the mayo and lemon juice as a topping, add salt and pepper to taste)	
4 ounces chopped cooked tilapia	Freebie
¼ cup mayonnaise	Freebie
1 tablespoon lemon juice	Freebie
¼ sliced avocado	Freebie
MEAL: Snack	
1 hard-cooked egg	Freebie
MEAL: Dinner (mix the greens, cheese, and vinegar as a side)	
3 ounces grilled steak	Freebie
2 cups spinach	Freebie
2 tablespoons feta cheese	Freebie
1 tablespoon balsamic vinegar	Freebie
MEAL: Dessert	
1 (5-ounce) glass red wine	14
DAILY TOTAL	**14 Sugar Calories**

MY WATER INTAKE
(8-ounce glasses):

1   2   3   4   5   6   7   8   More?

MY SLEEP QUALITY LAST NIGHT
(10 is highest):

1   2   3   4   5   6   7   8   9   10

MY ENERGY LEVEL YESTERDAY
(10 is highest):

1   2   3   4   5   6   7   8   9   10

☐ YOUR **WORKOUT**

BRIDGE AND PRESS
(x 3 minutes)

SUPINE KNEE TUCK
(x 2 minutes)

206

YOUR INCHES OFF! DAILY LOG

MEAL: Breakfast	SUGAR CALORIES (carb grams x 4)
½ cup cottage cheese	Freebie
2 tablespoons chopped pecans	Freebie
Coffee with half-and-half	Freebie
MEAL: Snack	
1 stick string cheese	Freebie
MEAL: Lunch (toss the ingredients with salt and pepper to taste)	
½ cup steamed chopped cauliflower	Freebie
½ cup steamed chopped broccoli	Freebie
2 tablespoons chopped red bell pepper	Freebie
3 slices chopped ham	Freebie
2 tablespoons olive oil	Freebie
MEAL: Snack	
5 celery sticks spread with cream cheese	Freebie
MEAL: Dinner	
3 ounces sliced cooked chicken breast	Freebie
2 cups mixed greens	Freebie
Olive oil and vinegar dressing	Freebie
Salt and pepper	Freebie
MEAL: Dessert	
1 (5-ounce) glass red wine	14
DAILY TOTAL	**14 Sugar Calories**

☐ YOUR **WORKOUT**

DEADLIFT AND ROW
(x 3 minutes)

STRAIGHT-ARM PLANK
(x 2 minutes)

MY WATER INTAKE
(8-ounce glasses):

1 2 3 4 5 6 7 8 More?

MY SLEEP QUALITY LAST NIGHT
(10 is highest):

1 2 3 4 5 6 7 8 9 10

MY ENERGY LEVEL YESTERDAY
(10 is highest):

1 2 3 4 5 6 7 8 9 10

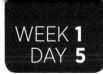

YOUR INCHES OFF! DAILY LOG

MEAL: Breakfast	SUGAR CALORIES (carb grams x 4)
2 poached eggs	Freebie
½ cup spinach	Freebie
2 strips turkey bacon	Freebie
MEAL: Snack	
¼ cup pumpkin seeds	Freebie
MEAL: Lunch (toss the ingredients together)	
5 medium shrimp	Freebie
2 cups shredded romaine	Freebie
5 cherry tomatoes	Freebie
2 tablespoons Caesar dressing	4
MEAL: Snack	
1 hard-cooked egg	Freebie
MEAL: Dinner (prepare as an open-faced burger)	
1 slice Food For Life Ezekiel 4:9 Sprouted Grain Bread	60
1 slice provolone	Freebie
3 ounces cooked lean ground beef patty	Freebie
1 tablespoon mustard	Freebie
¼ cup arugula	Freebie
MEAL: Dessert	
1 (5-ounce) glass red wine	14
DAILY TOTAL	**78 Sugar Calories**

MY WATER INTAKE
(8-ounce glasses):

1   2   3   4   5   6   7   8   More?

MY SLEEP QUALITY LAST NIGHT
(10 is highest):

1   2   3   4   5   6   7   8   9   10

MY ENERGY LEVEL YESTERDAY
(10 is highest):

1   2   3   4   5   6   7   8   9   10

☐ YOUR **WORKOUT**

BURPEE
(x 3 minutes)

CROSS-BODY HIGH KNEES
(x 2 minutes)

YOUR INCHES OFF! DAILY LOG

MEAL: Breakfast	SUGAR CALORIES (carb grams x 4)
½ cup cottage cheese	Freebie
2 tablespoons chopped pecans	Freebie
Coffee with half-and-half	Freebie
MEAL: Snack	
1 stick string cheese	Freebie
MEAL: Lunch (mix the mayo and lemon juice as a topping, add salt and pepper to taste)	
4 ounces chopped cooked tilapia	Freebie
¼ cup mayonnaise	Freebie
1 tablespoon lemon juice	Freebie
4 leaves romaine	Freebie
¼ sliced avocado	Freebie
MEAL: Snack	
5 celery sticks spread with cream cheese	Freebie
MEAL: Dinner (mix the greens, cheese, and vinegar as a side)	
3 ounces grilled steak	Freebie
2 cups spinach	Freebie
2 tablespoons feta cheese	Freebie
1 tablespoon balsamic vinegar	Freebie
MEAL: Dessert	
1 (5-ounce) glass red wine	14
DAILY TOTAL	**14 Sugar Calories**

☐ YOUR **WORKOUT**

OVERHEAD SWING
(x 3 minutes)

BIRD DOG
(x 2 minutes)

MY WATER INTAKE
(8-ounce glasses):
1 2 3 4 5 6 7 8 More?

MY SLEEP QUALITY LAST NIGHT
(10 is highest):
1 2 3 4 5 6 7 8 9 10

MY ENERGY LEVEL YESTERDAY
(10 is highest):
1 2 3 4 5 6 7 8 9 10

209

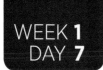

YOUR INCHES OFF! DAILY LOG

MEAL: Breakfast	SUGAR CALORIES (carb grams x 4)
2 poached eggs	Freebie
½ cup spinach	Freebie
2 strips turkey bacon	Freebie
MEAL: Snack	
¼ cup pumpkin seeds	Freebie
MEAL: Lunch (toss the ingredients with salt and pepper to taste)	
½ cup steamed chopped cauliflower	Freebie
½ cup steamed chopped broccoli	Freebie
2 tablespoons chopped red bell pepper	Freebie
3 slices chopped ham	Freebie
2 tablespoons olive oil	Freebie
MEAL: Snack	
1 hard-cooked egg	Freebie
MEAL: Dinner	
3 ounces sliced cooked chicken breast	Freebie
2 cups mixed greens	Freebie
Olive oil and vinegar dressing	Freebie
Salt and pepper	Freebie
MEAL: Dessert	
1 (5-ounce) glass red wine	14
DAILY TOTAL	**14 Sugar Calories**

MY WATER INTAKE
(8-ounce glasses):

1   2   3   4   5   6   7   8   More?

MY SLEEP QUALITY LAST NIGHT
(10 is highest):

1   2   3   4   5   6   7   8   9   10

MY ENERGY LEVEL YESTERDAY
(10 is highest):

1   2   3   4   5   6   7   8   9   10

IT'S **SUNDAY!**

You didn't have any exercises to do, but you should still be active and having fun. What did you do today?

_____

_____

_____

_____

YOUR INCHES OFF! DAILY LOG

MEAL: Breakfast	SUGAR CALORIES (carb grams x 4)
2 scrambled eggs	Freebie
2 tablespoons each chopped red bell pepper and onion	Freebie
2 tablespoons shredded pepper Jack cheese	Freebie
2 links breakfast sausage	Freebie
MEAL: Snack	
5 slices cucumber with 2 tablespoons feta cheese	Freebie
MEAL: Lunch (stack the first 4 ingredients in layers and drizzle with the vinegar)	
3 slices fresh mozzarella	Freebie
3 slices tomato	Freebie
3 strips cooked bacon	Freebie
3 leaves basil	Freebie
1 tablespoon balsamic vinegar	Freebie
MEAL: Snack	
2 slices Cheddar cheese	Freebie
MEAL: Dinner	
3 ounces grilled salmon	Freebie
2 cups spinach	Freebie
Olive oil and vinegar dressing	Freebie
MEAL: Dessert	
1 (5-ounce) glass red wine	14
DAILY TOTAL	**14 Sugar Calories**

☐ YOUR **WORKOUT**

SQUAT AND PRESS WITH WEIGHT
(x 3 minutes)

MOUNTAIN CLIMBERS
(x 2 minutes)

MY WATER INTAKE
(8-ounce glasses):

1 2 3 4 5 6 7 8 More?

MY SLEEP QUALITY LAST NIGHT
(10 is highest):

1 2 3 4 5 6 7 8 9 10

MY ENERGY LEVEL YESTERDAY
(10 is highest):

1 2 3 4 5 6 7 8 9 10

211

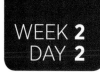
YOUR INCHES OFF! DAILY LOG

MEAL: Breakfast	SUGAR CALORIES (carb grams x 4)
1 sliced hard-cooked egg	Freebie
3 slices Cheddar cheese	Freebie
3 slices ham	Freebie
MEAL: Snack	
10 almonds	Freebie
MEAL: Lunch (toss the ingredients together)	
3 ounces sliced cooked chicken breast	Freebie
2 cups chopped romaine	Freebie
½ cucumber, sliced, and 5 cherry tomatoes	Freebie
2 tablespoons feta cheese	Freebie
2 tablespoons lemon juice, 1 tablespoon olive oil	Freebie
MEAL: Snack	
¼ cup pumpkin seeds	Freebie
MEAL: Dinner	
1 grilled pork chop	Freebie
1 cup sautéed broccoli	Freebie
1 cup sautéed mushrooms	Freebie
MEAL: Dessert	
1 (5-ounce) glass red wine	14
DAILY TOTAL	**14 Sugar Calories**

MY WATER INTAKE
(8-ounce glasses):

1 2 3 4 5 6 7 8 More?

MY SLEEP QUALITY LAST NIGHT
(10 is highest):

1 2 3 4 5 6 7 8 9 10

MY ENERGY LEVEL YESTERDAY
(10 is highest):

1 2 3 4 5 6 7 8 9 10

☐ YOUR **WORKOUT**

SUMO DEADLIFT HIGH PULL WITH WEIGHT
(x 3 minutes)

SIDE PLANK
(x 2 minutes)

YOUR INCHES OFF! DAILY LOG

MEAL: Breakfast	SUGAR CALORIES (carb grams x 4)
2 scrambled eggs	Freebie
2 tablespoons each chopped red bell pepper and onion	Freebie
2 tablespoons shredded pepper Jack cheese	Freebie
2 links breakfast sausage	Freebie
MEAL: Snack	
5 slices cucumber with 2 tablespoons feta cheese	Freebie
MEAL: Lunch (mix the ingredients, add salt and pepper to taste)	
1 can tuna	Freebie
2 tablespoons mayonnaise	Freebie
1 chopped scallion	Freebie
1 teaspoon lime juice	Freebie
MEAL: Snack	
2 slices Cheddar cheese	Freebie
MEAL: Dinner	
3 ounces sautéed chicken breast	Freebie
8 sautéed asparagus spears	Freebie
Salt and pepper	Freebie
MEAL: Dessert	
1 (5-ounce) glass red wine	14
DAILY TOTAL	**14 Sugar Calories**

☐ YOUR **WORKOUT**

BRIDGE AND PRESS WITH WEIGHT
(x 3 minutes)

CROSS-BODY MOUNTAIN CLIMBERS
(x 2 minutes)

MY WATER INTAKE
(8-ounce glasses):

1 2 3 4 5 6 7 8 More?

MY SLEEP QUALITY LAST NIGHT
(10 is highest):

1 2 3 4 5 6 7 8 9 10

MY ENERGY LEVEL YESTERDAY
(10 is highest):

1 2 3 4 5 6 7 8 9 10

213

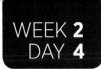
YOUR INCHES OFF! DAILY LOG

MEAL: Breakfast	SUGAR CALORIES (carb grams x 4)
1 sliced hard-cooked egg	Freebie
3 slices Cheddar cheese	Freebie
3 slices ham	Freebie
MEAL: Snack	
10 almonds	Freebie
MEAL: Lunch (stack the first 4 ingredients in layers and drizzle with the vinegar)	
3 slices fresh mozzarella	Freebie
3 slices tomato	Freebie
3 strips cooked bacon	Freebie
3 leaves basil	Freebie
1 tablespoon balsamic vinegar	Freebie
MEAL: Snack	
¼ cup sunflower seeds	Freebie
MEAL: Dinner	
3 ounces grilled salmon	Freebie
2 cups spinach	Freebie
Olive oil and vinegar dressing	Freebie
MEAL: Dessert	
1 (5-ounce) glass red wine	14
DAILY TOTAL	**14 Sugar Calories**

MY WATER INTAKE
(8-ounce glasses):

1   2   3   4   5   6   7   8   More?

MY SLEEP QUALITY LAST NIGHT
(10 is highest):

1   2   3   4   5   6   7   8   9   10

MY ENERGY LEVEL YESTERDAY
(10 is highest):

1   2   3   4   5   6   7   8   9   10

☐ YOUR **WORKOUT**

DEADLIFT AND ROW WITH WEIGHTS
(x 3 minutes)

STRAIGHT-ARM SIDE PLANK
(x 2 minutes)

YOUR INCHES OFF! DAILY LOG

MEAL: Breakfast	SUGAR CALORIES (carb grams x 4)
2 scrambled eggs	Freebie
2 tablespoons each chopped red bell pepper and onion	Freebie
2 tablespoons shredded pepper Jack cheese	Freebie
2 links breakfast sausage	Freebie
MEAL: Snack	
5 slices cucumber with 2 tablespoons feta cheese	Freebie
MEAL: Lunch (toss the ingredients together, add salt and pepper to taste)	
3 ounces sliced cooked chicken breast	Freebie
2 cups chopped romaine	Freebie
½ cucumber, sliced, and 5 cherry tomatoes	Freebie
2 tablespoons feta cheese	Freebie
2 tablespoons lemon juice, 1 tablespoon olive oil	Freebie
MEAL: Snack	
2 slices Cheddar cheese	Freebie
MEAL: Dinner	
1 grilled pork chop	Freebie
1 cup sautéed broccoli	Freebie
1 cup sautéed mushrooms	Freebie
MEAL: Dessert	
1 (5-ounce) glass red wine	14
DAILY TOTAL	**14 Sugar Calories**

☐ YOUR **WORKOUT**

BURPEE WITH PUSHUP
(x 3 minutes)

BIRD DOG WITH CRUNCH
(x 2 minutes)

MY WATER INTAKE
(8-ounce glasses):

1   2   3   4   5   6   7   8   More?

MY SLEEP QUALITY LAST NIGHT
(10 is highest):

1   2   3   4   5   6   7   8   9   10

MY ENERGY LEVEL YESTERDAY
(10 is highest):

1   2   3   4   5   6   7   8   9   10

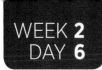
YOUR INCHES OFF! DAILY LOG

MEAL: Breakfast	SUGAR CALORIES (carb grams x 4)
1 sliced hard-cooked egg	Freebie
3 slices Cheddar cheese	Freebie
3 slices ham	Freebie
MEAL: Snack	
10 almonds	Freebie
MEAL: Lunch (mix the ingredients, add salt and pepper to taste)	
1 can tuna	Freebie
2 tablespoons mayonnaise	Freebie
1 chopped scallion	Freebie
1 teaspoon lime juice	Freebie
MEAL: Snack	
¼ cup sunflower seeds	Freebie
MEAL: Dinner	
3 ounces sautéed chicken breast	Freebie
8 sautéed asparagus spears	Freebie
Salt and pepper	Freebie
MEAL: Dessert	
1 (5-ounce) glass red wine	14
DAILY TOTAL	**14 Sugar Calories**

MY WATER INTAKE
(8-ounce glasses):

1   2   3   4   5   6   7   8   More?

MY SLEEP QUALITY LAST NIGHT
(10 is highest):

1   2   3   4   5   6   7   8   9   10

MY ENERGY LEVEL YESTERDAY
(10 is highest):

1   2   3   4   5   6   7   8   9   10

☐ YOUR **WORKOUT**

OVERHEAD SWING WITH WEIGHT
(x 3 minutes)

SUPINE STRAIGHT-LEG RAISE
(x 2 minutes)

YOUR INCHES OFF! DAILY LOG

MEAL: Breakfast	SUGAR CALORIES (carb grams x 4)
2 scrambled eggs	Freebie
2 tablespoons each chopped red bell pepper and onion	Freebie
2 tablespoons shredded pepper Jack cheese	Freebie
2 links breakfast sausage	Freebie
MEAL: Snack	
5 slices cucumber with 2 tablespoons feta cheese	Freebie
MEAL: Lunch (stack the first 4 ingredients in layers and drizzle with the vinegar)	
3 slices fresh mozzarella	Freebie
3 slices tomato	Freebie
3 strips cooked bacon	Freebie
3 leaves basil	Freebie
1 tablespoon balsamic vinegar	Freebie
MEAL: Snack	
2 slices Cheddar cheese	Freebie
MEAL: Dinner	
3 ounces grilled salmon	Freebie
2 cups spinach	Freebie
Olive oil and vinegar dressing	Freebie
MEAL: Dessert	
1 (5-ounce) glass red wine	14
DAILY TOTAL	**14 Sugar Calories**

IT'S **SUNDAY!**

You didn't have any exercises to do, but you should still be active and having fun. What did you do today?

_____

_____

_____

_____

_____

MY WATER INTAKE
(8-ounce glasses):

1   2   3   4   5   6   7   8   More?

MY SLEEP QUALITY LAST NIGHT
(10 is highest):

1   2   3   4   5   6   7   8   9   10

MY ENERGY LEVEL YESTERDAY
(10 is highest):

1   2   3   4   5   6   7   8   9   10

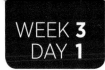

YOUR INCHES OFF! DAILY LOG

MEAL: Breakfast	SUGAR CALORIES (carb grams x 4)
2 eggs sunny-side up	Freebie
2 strips cooked bacon	Freebie
MEAL: Snack	
1 serving deli turkey	Freebie
MEAL: Lunch (the cucumber and feta can be a side or a topping)	
1 grilled hamburger patty	Freebie
3 slices cucumber	Freebie
2 tablespoons feta cheese	Freebie
Olive oil and vinegar (optional)	Freebie
Salt and pepper	Freebie
MEAL: Snack	
1 stick string cheese	Freebie
MEAL: Dinner (serve the first 3 ingredients on a bed of the spinach)	
1 sautéed halibut fillet	Freebie
¼ cup sautéed red bell pepper	Freebie
Salt and pepper	Freebie
2 cups spinach	Freebie
MEAL: Dessert	
1 (5-ounce) glass red wine	14
DAILY TOTAL	**14 Sugar Calories**

MY WATER INTAKE
(8-ounce glasses):

1   2   3   4   5   6   7   8   More?

MY SLEEP QUALITY LAST NIGHT
(10 is highest):

1   2   3   4   5   6   7   8   9   10

MY ENERGY LEVEL YESTERDAY
(10 is highest):

1   2   3   4   5   6   7   8   9   10

☐ YOUR **WORKOUT**

GLIDER LUNGE AND OVERHEAD LIFT
(x 3 minutes)

STANDING BAND PULL-APART
(x 2 minutes)

YOUR INCHES OFF! DAILY LOG

MEAL: Breakfast (combine the ingredients)	SUGAR CALORIES (carb grams x 4)
½ cup cottage cheese	Freebie
2 tablespoons chopped walnuts	Freebie
1 teaspoon unsweetened cocoa powder	Freebie
MEAL: Snack	
¼ cup macadamia nuts	Freebie
MEAL: Lunch (toss the ingredients with optional olive oil and vinegar)	
2 cups mixed greens	Freebie
¼ cup artichoke hearts	Freebie
2 tablespoons grated Parmesan	Freebie
3 ounces chopped cooked chicken breast	Freebie
MEAL: Snack	
1 hard-cooked egg	Freebie
MEAL: Dinner	
1 grilled steak	Freebie
1 cup cooked Brussels sprouts	Freebie
½ cup cooked mushrooms	Freebie
Salt and pepper	Freebie
MEAL: Dessert	
1 (5-ounce) glass red wine	14
DAILY TOTAL	**14 Sugar Calories**

☐ YOUR **WORKOUT**

SHOULDER-ELEVATED BRIDGE WITH PULL-APART
(x 3 minutes)

AROUND-THE-WORLD ELBOW PLANK
(x 2 minutes)

MY WATER INTAKE
(8-ounce glasses):

1 2 3 4 5 6 7 8 More?

MY SLEEP QUALITY LAST NIGHT
(10 is highest):

1 2 3 4 5 6 7 8 9 10

MY ENERGY LEVEL YESTERDAY
(10 is highest):

1 2 3 4 5 6 7 8 9 10

219

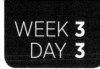
YOUR INCHES OFF! DAILY LOG

MEAL: Breakfast	SUGAR CALORIES (carb grams x 4)
2 eggs sunny-side up	Freebie
2 strips cooked bacon	Freebie
MEAL: Snack	
1 serving deli turkey	Freebie
MEAL: Lunch (serve the first 4 ingredients on a bed of the spinach)	
3 ounces baked chicken breast	Freebie
1 slice provolone	Freebie
¼ sliced avocado	Freebie
¼ chopped onion	Freebie
2 cups spinach	Freebie
MEAL: Snack	
1 stick string cheese	Freebie
MEAL: Dinner (combine the ingredients for a stir-fry)	
½ cup each sautéed onion and mushrooms	Freebie
1 minced sautéed clove garlic	Freebie
½ cup sautéed red bell pepper	Freebie
3 ounces ground sautéed turkey	Freebie
1 tablespoon soy sauce	Freebie
1 cup spinach	Freebie
MEAL: Dessert	
1 (5-ounce) glass red wine	14
DAILY TOTAL	**14 Sugar Calories**

MY WATER INTAKE
(8-ounce glasses):

1 2 3 4 5 6 7 8 More?

MY SLEEP QUALITY LAST NIGHT
(10 is highest):

1 2 3 4 5 6 7 8 9 10

MY ENERGY LEVEL YESTERDAY
(10 is highest):

1 2 3 4 5 6 7 8 9 10

☐ YOUR **WORKOUT**

SHORT-STEP BACKWARD LUNGE WITH SINGLE-ARM PRESS
(x 3 minutes)

RESISTANCE BAND PRESS-OUT
(x 2 minutes)

YOUR INCHES OFF! DAILY LOG

MEAL: Breakfast (combine the ingredients)	SUGAR CALORIES (carb grams x 4)
½ cup cottage cheese	Freebie
2 tablespoons chopped walnuts	Freebie
1 teaspoon unsweetened cocoa powder	Freebie
MEAL: Snack	
¼ cup macadamia nuts	Freebie
MEAL: Lunch (the cucumber and feta can be a side or a topping)	
1 grilled hamburger patty	Freebie
3 slices cucumber	Freebie
2 tablespoons feta cheese	Freebie
Olive oil and vinegar (optional)	Freebie
Salt and pepper	Freebie
MEAL: Snack	
1 hard-cooked egg	Freebie
MEAL: Dinner (serve the first 3 ingredients on a bed of the spinach)	
1 sautéed halibut fillet	Freebie
¼ cup sautéed red bell pepper	Freebie
Salt and pepper	Freebie
2 cups spinach	Freebie
MEAL: Dessert	
1 (5-ounce) glass red wine	14
DAILY TOTAL	**14 Sugar Calories**

☐ YOUR **WORKOUT**

SUPINE BRIDGE WITH GLIDER
(x 3 minutes)

**AROUND-THE-WORLD
ELBOW PLANK**
(x 2 minutes)

MY WATER INTAKE
(8-ounce glasses):

1   2   3   4   5   6   7   8   More?

MY SLEEP QUALITY LAST NIGHT
(10 is highest):

1   2   3   4   5   6   7   8   9   10

MY ENERGY LEVEL YESTERDAY
(10 is highest):

1   2   3   4   5   6   7   8   9   10

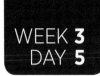

YOUR INCHES OFF! DAILY LOG

MEAL: Breakfast	SUGAR CALORIES (carb grams x 4)
2 eggs sunny-side up	Freebie
2 strips cooked bacon	Freebie
MEAL: Snack	
1 serving deli turkey	Freebie
MEAL: Lunch (toss the ingredients with optional olive oil and vinegar)	
2 cups mixed greens	Freebie
¼ cup artichoke hearts	Freebie
2 tablespoons grated Parmesan	Freebie
3 ounces chopped cooked chicken breast	Freebie
MEAL: Snack	
1 stick string cheese	Freebie
MEAL: Dinner	
1 grilled steak	Freebie
1 cup cooked Brussels sprouts	Freebie
½ cup cooked mushrooms	Freebie
Salt and pepper	Freebie
MEAL: Dessert	
1 (5-ounce) glass red wine	14
DAILY TOTAL	**14 Sugar Calories**

MY WATER INTAKE
(8-ounce glasses):

1   2   3   4   5   6   7   8   More?

MY SLEEP QUALITY LAST NIGHT
(10 is highest):

1   2   3   4   5   6   7   8   9   10

MY ENERGY LEVEL YESTERDAY
(10 is highest):

1   2   3   4   5   6   7   8   9   10

☐ YOUR **WORKOUT**

LONG-STEP LUNGE WITH OVERHEAD HOLD
(x 3 minutes)

CROSS-BODY WOOD CHOP
(x 2 minutes)

YOUR INCHES OFF! DAILY LOG

MEAL: Breakfast (combine the ingredients)	SUGAR CALORIES (carb grams x 4)
½ cup cottage cheese	Freebie
2 tablespoons chopped walnuts	Freebie
1 teaspoon unsweetened cocoa powder	Freebie
MEAL: Snack	
¼ cup macadamia nuts	Freebie
MEAL: Lunch (serve the first 4 ingredients on a bed of the spinach)	
3 ounces baked chicken breast	Freebie
1 slice provolone	Freebie
¼ sliced avocado	Freebie
¼ chopped onion	Freebie
2 cups spinach	Freebie
MEAL: Snack	
1 hard-cooked egg	Freebie
MEAL: Dinner (combine the ingredients with 1 tablespoon soy sauce for a stir-fry)	
½ cup each sautéed onion, mushrooms, red bell pepper	Freebie
1 minced sautéed clove garlic	Freebie
3 ounces ground sautéed turkey	Freebie
1 cup spinach	Freebie
MEAL: Dessert	
1 (5-ounce) glass red wine	14
DAILY TOTAL	**14 Sugar Calories**

☐ YOUR **WORKOUT**

BURPEE WITH OVERHEAD SWING
(x 3 minutes)

ALTERNATING LEG LIFT WITH PULL-APART
(x 2 minutes)

MY WATER INTAKE
(8-ounce glasses):

1   2   3   4   5   6   7   8   More?

MY SLEEP QUALITY LAST NIGHT
(10 is highest):

1   2   3   4   5   6   7   8   9   10

MY ENERGY LEVEL YESTERDAY
(10 is highest):

1   2   3   4   5   6   7   8   9   10

YOUR INCHES OFF! DAILY LOG

	SUGAR CALORIES (carb grams x 4)
MEAL: Breakfast	
2 eggs sunny-side up	Freebie
2 strips cooked bacon	Freebie
MEAL: Snack	
1 serving deli turkey	Freebie
MEAL: Lunch (the cucumber and feta can be a side or a topping)	
1 grilled hamburger patty	Freebie
3 slices cucumber	Freebie
2 tablespoons feta cheese	Freebie
Olive oil and vinegar (optional)	Freebie
Salt and pepper	Freebie
MEAL: Snack	
1 stick string cheese	Freebie
MEAL: Dinner (serve the first 3 ingredients on a bed of the spinach)	
1 sautéed halibut fillet	Freebie
¼ cup sautéed red bell pepper	Freebie
Salt and pepper	Freebie
2 cups spinach	Freebie
MEAL: Dessert	
1 (5-ounce) glass red wine	14
DAILY TOTAL	**14 Sugar Calories**

MY WATER INTAKE
(8-ounce glasses):

1   2   3   4   5   6   7   8   More?

MY SLEEP QUALITY LAST NIGHT
(10 is highest):

1   2   3   4   5   6   7   8   9   10

MY ENERGY LEVEL YESTERDAY
(10 is highest):

1   2   3   4   5   6   7   8   9   10

IT'S **SUNDAY!**

You didn't have any exercises to do, but you should still be active and having fun. What did you do today?

_____
_____
_____
_____
_____

YOUR INCHES OFF! DAILY LOG

MEAL: Breakfast (combine the ingredients as an omelet)	SUGAR CALORIES (carb grams x 4)
2 eggs	Freebie
¼ cup Mexican cheese blend	Freebie
2 tablespoons salsa	Freebie
¼ sliced avocado	Freebie
MEAL: Snack	
1 serving deli ham	Freebie
MEAL: Lunch	
3 ounces panfried chicken	Freebie
1 tablespoon Dijon mustard	Freebie
1 chopped sautéed zucchini	Freebie
MEAL: Snack	
¼ cup pecans	Freebie
MEAL: Dinner (toss the veggies, cheese, and dressing as a side)	
1 grilled flank steak	Freebie
2 cups spinach	Freebie
5 sliced cherry tomatoes	Freebie
2 tablespoons feta cheese	Freebie
Olive oil and vinegar dressing	Freebie
MEAL: Dessert	
1 (5-ounce) glass red wine	14
DAILY TOTAL	**14 Sugar Calories**

☐ YOUR **WORKOUT**

GOBLET GLIDER LUNGE
(x 3 minutes)

HIGH KNEES WITH OVERHEAD HOLD
(x 2 minutes)

MY WATER INTAKE
(8-ounce glasses):

1 2 3 4 5 6 7 8 More?

MY SLEEP QUALITY LAST NIGHT
(10 is highest):

1 2 3 4 5 6 7 8 9 10

MY ENERGY LEVEL YESTERDAY
(10 is highest):

1 2 3 4 5 6 7 8 9 10

225

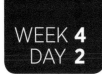
YOUR INCHES OFF! DAILY LOG

MEAL: Breakfast	SUGAR CALORIES (carb grams x 4)
1 cup plain Greek yogurt	Freebie
2 tablespoons blackberries	11
MEAL: Snack	
5 celery sticks dipped in mustard	Freebie
MEAL: Lunch (combine the ingredients)	
2 cups shredded romaine	Freebie
4 slices deli turkey, chopped	Freebie
1 chopped hard-cooked egg	Freebie
2 tablespoons blue cheese crumbles	Freebie
2 tablespoons blue cheese dressing	Freebie
MEAL: Snack	
1 slice provolone	Freebie
MEAL: Dinner	
1 grilled salmon fillet	Freebie
1 cup arugula	Freebie
¼ cup sautéed zucchini	Freebie
Lemon juice	Freebie
Salt and pepper	Freebie
MEAL: Dessert	
1 (5-ounce) glass red wine	14
DAILY TOTAL	**25 Sugar Calories**

MY WATER INTAKE
(8-ounce glasses):

1   2   3   4   5   6   7   8   More?

MY SLEEP QUALITY LAST NIGHT
(10 is highest):

1   2   3   4   5   6   7   8   9   10

MY ENERGY LEVEL YESTERDAY
(10 is highest):

1   2   3   4   5   6   7   8   9   10

☐ YOUR **WORKOUT**

SUMO DEADLIFT WITH JUMP
(x 3 minutes)

LEG LIFT WITH BAND STRETCH
(x 2 minutes)

YOUR INCHES OFF! DAILY LOG

MEAL: Breakfast (combine the ingredients as an omelet)	SUGAR CALORIES (carb grams x 4)
2 eggs	Freebie
¼ cup Mexican cheese blend	Freebie
2 tablespoons salsa	Freebie
¼ sliced avocado	Freebie
MEAL: Snack	
1 serving deli ham	Freebie
MEAL: Lunch (combine the first 3 ingredients and serve on the romaine)	
12 cooked baby shrimp	Freebie
1 teaspoon each lime juice and finely chopped dill	Freebie
1 tablespoon mayonnaise	Freebie
3 leaves romaine	Freebie
MEAL: Snack	
¼ cup pecans	Freebie
MEAL: Dinner (toss the ingredients with a balsamic vinegar dressing)	
1 cup each chopped spinach and romaine	Freebie
1 chopped tomato	Freebie
2 chopped hard-cooked eggs	Freebie
3 ounces sliced cooked chicken breast	Freebie
MEAL: Dessert	
1 (5-ounce) glass red wine	14
DAILY TOTAL	**14 Sugar Calories**

☐ YOUR **WORKOUT**

**LATERAL GLIDER LUNGE
WITH WEIGHT**
(x 3 minutes)

TORSO TWIST WITH WEIGHT
(x 2 minutes)

MY WATER INTAKE
(8-ounce glasses):

1   2   3   4   5   6   7   8   More?

MY SLEEP QUALITY LAST NIGHT
(10 is highest):

1   2   3   4   5   6   7   8   9   10

MY ENERGY LEVEL YESTERDAY
(10 is highest):

1   2   3   4   5   6   7   8   9   10

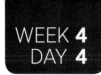
YOUR INCHES OFF! DAILY LOG

MEAL: Breakfast	SUGAR CALORIES (carb grams x 4)
1 cup plain Greek yogurt	Freebie
2 tablespoons blackberries	11
MEAL: Snack	
5 celery sticks dipped in mustard	Freebie
MEAL: Lunch	
3 ounces panfried chicken	Freebie
1 tablespoon Dijon mustard	Freebie
1 chopped sautéed zucchini	Freebie
MEAL: Snack	
1 slice provolone	Freebie
MEAL: Dinner (toss the veggies, cheese, and dressing as a side)	
1 grilled flank steak	Freebie
2 cups spinach	Freebie
5 sliced cherry tomatoes	Freebie
2 tablespoons feta cheese	Freebie
Olive oil and vinegar dressing	Freebie
MEAL: Dessert	
1 (5-ounce) glass red wine	14
DAILY TOTAL	**25 Sugar Calories**

MY WATER INTAKE
(8-ounce glasses):

1   2   3   4   5   6   7   8   More?

MY SLEEP QUALITY LAST NIGHT
(10 is highest):

1   2   3   4   5   6   7   8   9   10

MY ENERGY LEVEL YESTERDAY
(10 is highest):

1   2   3   4   5   6   7   8   9   10

☐ YOUR **WORKOUT**

SINGLE-LEG BALANCE TOUCH
(x 3 minutes)

SINGLE-ARM PLANK
(x 2 minutes)

YOUR INCHES OFF! DAILY LOG

MEAL: Breakfast (combine the ingredients as an omelet)	SUGAR CALORIES (carb grams x 4)
2 eggs	Freebie
¼ cup Mexican cheese blend	Freebie
2 tablespoons salsa	Freebie
¼ sliced avocado	Freebie
MEAL: Snack	
1 serving deli ham	Freebie
MEAL: Lunch (combine the ingredients)	
2 cups shredded romaine	Freebie
4 slices deli turkey, chopped	Freebie
1 chopped hard-cooked egg	Freebie
2 tablespoons blue cheese crumbles	Freebie
2 tablespoons blue cheese dressing	Freebie
MEAL: Snack	
¼ cup pecans	Freebie
MEAL: Dinner	
1 grilled salmon fillet	Freebie
1 cup arugula	Freebie
¼ cup sautéed zucchini	Freebie
MEAL: Dessert	
1 (5-ounce) glass red wine	14
DAILY TOTAL	**14 Sugar Calories**

☐ YOUR **WORKOUT**

BURPEE WITH WEIGHT
(x 3 minutes)

HIGH KNEES WITH OVERHEAD HOLD
(x 2 minutes)

MY WATER INTAKE
(8-ounce glasses):
1   2   3   4   5   6   7   8   More?

MY SLEEP QUALITY LAST NIGHT
(10 is highest):
1   2   3   4   5   6   7   8   9   10

MY ENERGY LEVEL YESTERDAY
(10 is highest):
1   2   3   4   5   6   7   8   9   10

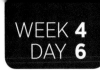
YOUR INCHES OFF! DAILY LOG

MEAL: Breakfast	SUGAR CALORIES (carb grams x 4)
1 cup plain Greek yogurt	Freebie
2 tablespoons blackberries	11
MEAL: Snack	
5 celery sticks dipped in mustard	Freebie
MEAL: Lunch (combine the first 3 ingredients and serve on the romaine)	
12 cooked baby shrimp	Freebie
1 teaspoon each lime juice and finely chopped dill	Freebie
1 tablespoon mayonnaise	Freebie
3 leaves romaine	Freebie
MEAL: Snack	
¼ cup pecans	Freebie
MEAL: Dinner (toss the ingredients with a balsamic vinegar dressing)	
1 cup each chopped spinach and romaine	Freebie
1 chopped tomato	Freebie
2 chopped hard-cooked eggs	Freebie
3 ounces sliced cooked chicken breast	Freebie
MEAL: Dessert	
1 (5-ounce) glass red wine	14
DAILY TOTAL	**25 Sugar Calories**

MY WATER INTAKE
(8-ounce glasses):

1   2   3   4   5   6   7   8   More?

MY SLEEP QUALITY LAST NIGHT
(10 is highest):

1   2   3   4   5   6   7   8   9   10

MY ENERGY LEVEL YESTERDAY
(10 is highest):

1   2   3   4   5   6   7   8   9   10

☐ YOUR **WORKOUT**

SINGLE-LEG BALANCE WITH ONE-ARM ROW
(x 3 minutes)

SINGLE-ARM PLANK WITH ROTATION
(x 2 minutes)

YOUR INCHES OFF! DAILY LOG

MEAL: Breakfast (combine the ingredients as an omelet)	SUGAR CALORIES (carb grams x 4)
2 eggs	Freebie
¼ cup Mexican cheese blend	Freebie
2 tablespoons salsa	Freebie
¼ sliced avocado	Freebie
MEAL: Snack	
1 serving deli ham	Freebie
MEAL: Lunch	
3 ounces panfried chicken	Freebie
1 tablespoon Dijon mustard	Freebie
1 chopped sautéed zucchini	Freebie
MEAL: Snack	
¼ cup pecans	Freebie
MEAL: Dinner (toss the veggies, cheese, and dressing as a side)	
1 grilled flank steak	Freebie
2 cups spinach	Freebie
5 sliced cherry tomatoes	Freebie
2 tablespoons feta cheese	Freebie
Olive oil and vinegar dressing	Freebie
MEAL: Dessert	
1 (5-ounce) glass red wine	14
DAILY TOTAL	**14 Sugar Calories**

IT'S **SUNDAY!**

You didn't have any exercises to do, but you should still be active and having fun. What did you do today?

_____
_____
_____
_____
_____

MY WATER INTAKE
(8-ounce glasses):

1 2 3 4 5 6 7 8 More?

MY SLEEP QUALITY LAST NIGHT
(10 is highest):

1 2 3 4 5 6 7 8 9 10

MY ENERGY LEVEL YESTERDAY
(10 is highest):

1 2 3 4 5 6 7 8 9 10

231

ACKNOWLEDGMENTS

I owe particular gratitude to my amazing team, without whom nothing would be possible. To my incredible fitness developer and dear friend, Stephen Steigler—your contributions to the book were truly invaluable. You are a perfect example of living this lifestyle and you are a true inspiration. To Kristin Penne, for keeping us organized, on time, and sane. Your support and assistance mean so much. To Oliver Stephenson, for your direction and support. I couldn't do it without you. You truly know how to apply your incredible commitment and talent to our mission. You make it all run! To Marianne McGinnis, your hard work and dedication mean so much. Thank you for all you do.

A huge, heartfelt thank-you to the whole Rodale Team. To Mike Zimmerman, without your hard work, dedication, and commitment, this project would not have been possible. To Mary Ann Naples, Anne Egan, Elizabeth Neal, Yelena Gitlin Nesbit, Emily Weber, Brent Gallenberger, and most especially to my dear friend Maria Rodale, for always believing in me. Thank you all for your belief in this project and your hard work to make it come to life.

A very special thank-you to my invaluable circle of experts: Gary Taubes, Dr. Robert Lustig, Dr. Mehmet Oz, Dr. Nicholas Perricone, Dr. Christiane Northrup, Dr. David Ludwig, Michael Pollan, Dr. Vincent Pedre, and Dr. Andrew Weil.

To my clients who have broken free from conventional wisdom and have finally reached their goal weight by working smarter, not harder—you all inspire me each and every day.

I wish to thank so many others who have contributed to this book as well as my overall vision and mission. Their advice, knowledge, and support have been so valuable, and I would not be where I am today without them. I wish to thank a few of them here.

- Abra Potkin
- Al Roker
- Alexandra Cohen
- Allison Markowitz
- Andy Jenkins
- Anthony Robbins
- Bill Geddie
- Blair Atkins
- Bob Wietrak
- Bobbi Brown
- Bobby Flay
- Bruce Barlean
- Carol Brooks
- Cathy Chermol
- Chef Art Smith
- Chef Emeril Lagasse
- Chris Hendrickson
- Clate Mask
- Daniel Sheldon
- David Thomsen
- Diane Sawyer
- Dustin Nigilo
- Eben Pagan
- Evan Dollard
- Frank Kern
- Ginnie Roeglin
- Hanna Richert
- Heather Spangler
- Hillary Estey McLoughlin
- Howard Bragman
- Jacqui Stafford
- Janet Annino
- Jaireck Robbins
- Jared Davis
- Jay Robb
- Joanna Parides
- Joe Fusco
- John Redmann
- Jon Davidson
- Jose Pretlow
- Joseph Pappa
- Joseph Quesada
- Katie Couric
- Kelly Ripa
- Kenny Rueter
- Kirk Masters
- Lance Bass & the Dirty Pop Team @ Sirius Satellite Radio
- Leslie Marcus
- Linda Fennell
- Lisa Gregorisch-Dempsey
- Louise Hay
- Maggie Jaqua
- Marc Victor
- Mario Batali
- Mark Sisson
- Marta Fox
- Martha Stewart
- Mary-Ellen Keating
- Maura Wogan
- Mel Maurer
- Michael Koenings
- Michelle McGowen
- Natalie Morales
- Oprah Winfrey
- Pennie Ianniciello
- President Bill Clinton
- Preston Stapley
- Rachael Ray
- Richard Galanti
- Richard Heller
- Robbie McMillin
- Robin Mead
- Robin Roberts
- Sage Robbins
- Scott Eason
- Scott Martineau
- Sheryl Underwood
- Suzanne Somers
- Suze Orman
- Terence Noonan
- Tim Austgen
- Tom Blair
- Toni Richi
- Travis Rosser
- Wayne Dyer
- Wioleta Gramek

INDEX

Index

Foam rolling
  exercises (*cont.*)
    Quadricep-and-Hip-
      Flexor Roll, 148, **148**
    Shoulder-Blade Roll, 151, **151**
    Upper-Back Roll, 150, **150**
  health benefits of, 144
Focus words, 22
Food label, **160**
Foods, 157. *See also* Diet; Freebie
  Foods; *specific type*
Ford, Henry, 39
Form of exercises, maintaining, 21
Freebie Foods
  dairy products, 173–74
  defining, 158
  dietary fat, 173
  eggs, 159
  flours, 170
  fruits, 159
  herbs, 172
  Inches Off! Your Tummy
    eating program and,
    158–60, 158
  other, 174
  protein, 169–71
  spices, 172
  tomatoes, 159
  vegetables, 158
  weight loss and, 160
Friends and weight loss, 189, 191
Frozen foods, 179
Fruits, 157, 159, 177

G

Gandhi, Mahatma, 95
Grab-and-go foods, 166
Grains, 175–76
Greek yogurt, 157

H

Happiness, 13, 190
Health, beliefs about, xv
Herbs, 172

High-intensity interval training
  (HIIT), 9–10
Hunger, 188
Hunter-gather lifestyle, 1–2, 2
Hydration, 161, 200

I

Inches Off! Your Tummy eating
    plan. *See also* Freebie
    Foods; Sugar Calories
  design of, 159
  desserts and, 160
  5-Minute Fitness Formula
    and, 157–58
  Freebie Foods and, 158–60,
    158
  meal planner, sample, 154,
    161
  principles of, 153
  protein in, 158
  safety belt system and
    audiotape, 164–65
    grab-and-go foods, 166
    jorgecruise.com Web site
      or Facebook, 166–67
    poster, before-and-after,
    166
    purpose of, 164
    quotations, 165–66
    selecting three, 167, 167
  water and, 159
Inches Off! Your Tummy
    program. *See also* Five-
    Minute Fitness
    Formula; *specific week
    number*
  calories burned by, 5
  caution about, 17, 24
  components of, 5
  continuing, 25, 183
  design of, xiv, 3, 5, 9
  equipment, **20**, 20
  5-minute fitness routine and,
    21
    adding to, 24
  form of exercises and, 21

health benefits of, 12–13, 16
impact of, 16–17
motivation for, 22
rest and, 23
stats before starting,
  recording, 31
time required for, xiv, 5–7, 9
tips, 21, 22–23
workout overview, 19
Information, correct weight-
  loss, xiii-xiv
Insulin, 155, 158
Intensity of exercise, 2–3, 6, 10
Interval exercise, 6, 9–10, 14

J

Joint stability, *12*
jorgecruise.com Web site or
    Facebook, 154, 166–67

L

Label, food, **160**
Laborsaving devices, avoiding,
    201
Lady Gaga, 107
Lamb, 171
Lean Cuisine frozen meals,
    179
Legumes, 175
Lewis, C. S., 18
Lifestyle
  changes, making long-
    lasting, xii-xiv, 193
  modern, 1–3
  sedentary, 14–15, 17
Light sources, sleeping and
    waking and, 197, 200
Lycopene, 159

M

Mansfield, Jayne, 103
Marshall, Peter, 119

Index

Index